Encyclopedic Dictionary of AIDS-Related Terminology

Encylopedic Dictionary of AIDS-Related Terminology

Jeffrey T. Huber, PhD
Mary L. Gillaspy, MLS, MS

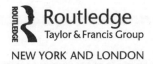

Routledge
Taylor & Francis Group

NEW YORK AND LONDON

First Published by

The Haworth Information Press, an imprint of The Haworth Press, Inc., 10 Alice Street, Binghamton, NY 13904-1580

Transferred to digital printing in 2011 by Routledge
711 Third Avenue, New York, NY 10017
2 Park Square, Milton Park, Abingdon, Oxon, OX14 4RN

This publication is a second edition of *Dictionary of AIDS-Related Terminology,* published by Neal-Schuman Publishers, Inc., 1993.

Cover design by Monica L. Seifert.

Library of Congress Cataloging-in-Publication Data

Huber, Jeffrey T.
    Encyclopedic dictionary of AIDS-related terminology / Jeffrey T. Huber, Mary L. Gillaspy.
      p.   cm.
    ISBN 0-7890-0714-2 (hard : alk. paper)—ISBN 0-7890-1207-3 (soft : alk. paper)
    1. AIDS (Disease)—Dictionaries. I. Gillaspy, Mary L. II. Title

RC607.A26 H8955 2000
616.97′92—dc21

                                            00-038919

ACKNOWLEDGMENT

The authors gratefully acknowledge the assistance of Jana K. Kastelhun for technical support.

ABOUT THE AUTHORS

Jeffrey T. Huber, PhD, is Assistant Professor at the School of Library and Information Studies at Texas Woman's University in Denton. He has more than ten years of experience working in the HIV/AIDS arena and is a recognized authority concerning this body of knowledge. Dr. Huber has published several books focusing on HIV/AIDS as well as numerous articles and presentations.

Mary L. Gillaspy, MLS, MS, has worked in the AIDS arena for more than ten years. She was the first librarian at the AIDS Resource Center in Dallas, Texas, and has continued to work with AIDS patients and caregivers in consumer health librarian positions at the University of Texas M. D. Anderson Cancer Center in Houston, and at Northwestern Memorial Hospital in Chicago, Illinois.

Introduction

The terminology associated with the acquired immunodeficiency syndrome (AIDS) and the human immunodeficiency virus (HIV) continues expanding in proportion to the proliferation of information currently available regarding the epidemic. In addition to existing terms, the pandemic has created its own vernacular. This work seeks to detail generally accepted meanings for the various words and phrases found in discussions of the interdisciplinary aspects of the pandemic. AIDS and HIV include medical, legal, social, psychological, and religious issues. Individuals from most socioeconomic backgrounds and organizations operating at the local, state, national, and international levels have been involved in the fight to stop the spread of the disease. As the epidemic continues to grow, it is expected that the complex nature of the verbiage associated with it will be further complicated.

This work, *Encyclopedic Dictionary of AIDS-Related Terminology*, provides an alphabetical list and explanation of key words, names, and phrases generally found in discussions of AIDS and HIV. The dictionary includes abbreviations, acronyms, historical terms, medical terminology, drugs associated with past and present therapy, major organizations and institutions, and AIDS-specific sources of information. Dates, histories, addresses, telephone numbers, and Web sites are included where appropriate and when available. Cross-references are provided from abbreviations, acronyms, vernacular, and product names to the main entry for the appropriate heading.

Since the acquired immunodeficiency syndrome and the human immunodeficiency virus involve many complex issues from a variety of disciplines, and given that the epidemic is in a constant state of flux, this work should not be construed as a comprehensive listing of every term, source of information, or organization associated with the epidemic. Rather, it is a presentation of the more common verbiage included in discussions of AIDS and HIV. For terms not included in this work, users should consider other sources of information such as *Dorland's Illustrated Medical Dictionary, The HIV Drug Book, Stedman's Medical Dictionary, Taber's Cyclopedic Medical Dictionary, The United States Government Manual,* or *Webster's New World Dictionary.*

REFERENCES

Dorland's Illustrated Medical Dictionary, Twenty-eighth Edition. Philadelphia, W.B. Saunders Co., 1994.

Kearny, Brian. *The HIV Drug Book.* New York: Pocket Books, 1995.

Stedman's Medical Dictionary, Twenty-sixth Edition. Baltimore: Williams & Wilkins, 1995.

Taber's Cyclopedic Medical Dictionary, Seventeenth Edition. Philadelphia: F.A. Davis, 1993.

The United States Government Manual. Washington, DC: Office of the Federal Register, National Archives and Records Service, General Services Administration: For sale by the Supt. of Docs., U.S. G.P.O., 1973- .

Webster's New World Dictionary of American English, Third College Edition. New York: Prentice-Hall.

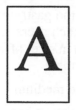

AAPHR: *See* AMERICAN ASSOCIATION OF PHYSICIANS FOR HUMAN RIGHTS.

abacavir: Nucleoside reverse transcriptase inhibitor, designed to be used in combination with other anti-retroviral drugs. The trade name is Ziagen. *See also* NON-NUCLEOSIDE REVERSE TRANSCRIPTASE INHIBITOR.

Abbott Laboratories: A pharmaceutical company located in North Chicago, Illinois. Among its many other products, Abbott manufactures the antibody test to detect the presence of the human immunodeficiency virus. It also produces numerous educational materials concerning HIV and AIDS. Abbott Laboratories, 100 Abbott Park Rd., Abbott Park, IL 60064-3500. Telephone: (847) 937-6100.

Abelcet: *See* AMPHOTERICIN B.

abortion: The voluntary, premature termination of pregnancy. The legal definition as to the point at which the fetus is capable of living outside of the uterus varies from state to state, but is usually considered to be 20-24 weeks or greater than 500 grams. Symptoms commonly experienced during abortions include uterine contractions, uterine hemorrhage (sometimes including tissue), dilation of the cervix, and ejection of fetal material.

abscess: A localized collection of pus resulting from the displacement or disintegration of tissue in any part of the body.

abstinence: (1) Voluntarily refraining from a particular behavior, such as engaging in sexual activities. (2) A safe sex technique whereby individuals voluntarily refrain from engaging in sexual activities. *See also* SAFE SEX.

accelerated approval: Regulatory mechanism established by the Food and Drug Administration in an effort to speed products to market for HIV disease, some cancers, and other deadly diseases. Early approval is based on laboratory markers (e.g., increased CD4 counts) rather than clinical endpoints, such as a longer lifespan following infection.

ACF: *See* ADMINISTRATION FOR CHILDREN AND FAMILIES.

ACHA *See* AMERICAN COLLEGE HEALTH ASSOCIATION.

achlorhydria: (1) The absence of hydrochloric acid in the gastric juices. (2) The absence of hydrochloric acid in the stomach secretions; a result of the atrophy (wasting away or diminution in size) of the gastric mucous membrane. *Also called* GASTRIC ANACIDITY.

acidophil: A bacterial organism that grows well in an acid medium.

acidophilus: Bacteria most commonly found in yogurt that, when ingested, helps restore "good" bacteria that are essential for the digestive process, yet may be compromised or even eliminated by antibiotics taken either indiscriminately or over a long period of time. Also promotes the prevention of candidiasis, or thrush.

acidophilus milk: Milk fermented by lactobacillus acidophilus cultures. It is used to modify the bacterial flora of the digestive tract and works as an intestinal cleanser. Acidophilus also helps prevent fungus, diverticulosis, acne, and bad breath. It helps in the absorption of calcium as well as other minerals.

ACIDS: *See* ACQUIRED COMMUNITY IMMUNE DEFICIENCY SYNDROME.

ACLU: *See* AMERICAN CIVIL LIBERTIES UNION.

acquired community immune deficiency syndrome (ACIDS): One of a group of names initially used to denote the acquired immunodeficiency syndrome. The current nomenclature was adopted in 1981. *See also* COMMUNITY ACQUIRED IMMUNE DEFICIENCY SYNDROME, GAY-RELATED IMMUNE DEFICIENCY, and ACQUIRED IMMUNODEFICIENCY SYNDROME.

acquired immune deficiency syndrome: *See* ACQUIRED IMMUNODEFICIENCY SYNDROME.

acquired immunodeficiency syndrome (AIDS): (1) Illness characterized by infection with the human immunodeficiency virus (HIV) coupled with the presence of one or more of a constellation of opportunistic infections or diseases (e.g., *Pneumocystis carinii* pneumonia, Kaposi's sarcoma, candidiasis, etc.) and the absence of any other known cause of immunodeficiency. AIDS does not include all manifestations of HIV-related illnesses. (2) The Centers for Disease Control and Prevention currently defines AIDS to include all HIV-infected persons with CD4+ T-lymphocyte counts of

<200 cells/cubic millimeter or a CD4+ percentage of <14. In addition to retaining the 23 clinical conditions in the previous AIDS surveillance definition, the expanded definition includes pulmonary tuberculosis (TB), recurrent pneumonia, and invasive cervical cancer. This expanded definition requires laboratory confirmation of HIV infection in persons with a CD4+ T-lymphocyte count of <200 cells/cubic millimeter or with one of the added clinical conditions. This expanded definition for reporting cases to the CDC became effective January 1, 1993.

EQUIVALENCES FOR ABSOLUTE NUMBERS OF CD4+

T lymphocytes and CD4+ Percentage*

CD4+ T cell category	CD4+ T cells/cubic millimeter	CD4 = percentage (%)
(1)	≥ 500	≥ 29
(2)	200-499	14-28
(3)	< 200	< 14

CONDITIONS INCLUDED IN THE 1993 AIDS SURVEILLANCE CASE DEFINITION

- Candidiasis of bronchi, trachea, or lungs
- Candidiasis, esophageal
- Cervical cancer, invasive**
- Coccidioidomycosis, disseminated or extrapulmonary
- Cryptococcosis, extrapulmonary
- Cryptosporidiosis, chronic intestinal (>1 month's duration)
- Cytomegalovirus disease (other than liver, spleen, or nodes)
- Cytomegalovirus retinitis (with loss of vision)
- Encephalopathy, HIV-related
- Herpes simplex: chronic ulcer(s) (>1 month's duration);
  or bronchitis, pneumonitis, or esophagitis

---

*The percentage of lymphocytes that are CD4+ cells.
**Added in the 1993 expansion of the AIDS surveillance case definition.

- Histoplasmosis, disseminated or extrapulmonary
- Isosporiasis, chronic intestinal (>1 month's duration)
- Kaposi's sarcoma
- Lymphoma, Burkitt's (or equivalent term)
- Lymphoma, immunoblastic (or equivalent term)
- Lymphoma, primary, of brain
- *Mycobacterium avium* complex or *M. kansasii*, disseminated or extrapulmonary
- *Mycobacterium tuberculosis*, any site (pulmonary* or extrapulmonary)
- *Pneumocystis carinii* pneumonia
- Pneumonia, recurrent*
- Progressive multifocal leukoencephalopathy
- *Salmonella* septicemia, recurrent
- Toxoplasmosis of brain
- Wasting syndrome due to HIV

DEFINITIVE DIAGNOSTIC METHODS
FOR DISEASES INDICATIVE OF AIDS

Diseases	Diagnostic Methods
Cryptosporidiosis	Microscopy (histology or cytology)
Isosporiasis	
Kaposi's sarcoma	
Lymphoma	
Pneumocystis carinii pneumonia	
Progressive multifocal leukoencephalopathy	
Toxoplasmosis	
Cervical cancer	
Candidiasis	Gross inspection by endoscopy or autopsy, or by microscopy (histology or cytology) on a specimen obtained directly from the tissues affected (including scraping from the mucosal surface), not from a culture.

*Added in the 1993 expansion of the AIDS surveillance case definition.

Diseases	Diagnostic Methods
Coccidioidomycosis	Microscopy (histology or cytology), culture, or detection of antigen in a specimen obtained directly from the tissues affected or a fluid from those tissues.
Cryptococcosis	
Cytomegalovirus	
Herpes simplex virus	
Histoplasmosis	
Tuberculosis	Culture
Other mycobacteriosis	
Salmonellosis	
HIV encephalopathy (dementia)	Clinical findings of disabling cognitive or motor dysfunction interfering with occupation or activities of daily living, progressing over weeks to months, in the absence of a concurrent illness or condition other than HIV infection that could explain the findings. Methods to rule out such concurrent illnesses and conditions must include cerebrospinal fluid examination and either brain imaging (computed tomography or magnetic resonance) or autopsy.
HIV wasting syndrome	Findings of profound involuntary weight loss of >10 percent of baseline body weight plus either chronic diarrhea (at least two loose stools per day for ≥ 30 days), or chronic weakness and documented fever (for ≥ 30 days, intermittent or constant in the absence of a concurrent illness or condition other than HIV infection that could explain the findings (e.g., cancer, tuberculosis, cryptosporidiosis, or other specific enteritis).
Pneumonia, recurrent	Recurrent (more than one episode in a one-year period), acute (new X ray evidence not present earlier) pneumonia diagnosed by both: (a) culture (or other organism-specific

Diseases	Diagnostic Methods
	diagnostic method) obtained from a clinically reliable specimen of a pathogen that typically causes pneumonia (other than *Pneumocystis carinii* or *Mycobacterium tuberculosis*), and (b) radiologic evidence of pneumonia; cases that do not have laboratory confirmation of a causative organism for one of the episodes of pneumonia will be considered as presumptively diagnosed.

SUGGESTED GUIDELINES FOR PRESUMPTIVE DIAGNOSIS OF DISEASE INDICATIVE OF AIDS

Diseases	Presumptive Criteria
Candidiasis of esophagus	a. Recent onset of retrosternal pain of swallowing; AND

b. Oral candidiasis diagnosed by the gross appearance of white patches or plaques on an erythematous base or by the microscopic appearance of fungal mycelial filaments from a noncultured specimen scraped from the oral mucosa. |
| Cytomegalovirus retinitis | A characteristic appearance on serial ophthalmoscopic examinations (e.g., discrete patches of retinal whitening with distinct borders, spreading in a centrifugal manner along the paths of blood vessels, progressing over several months, and frequently associated with retinal vasculitis, hemorrhage, and necrosis).

Resolution of active disease leaves retinal scarring and atrophy with retinal pigment epithelial mottling. |
| Mycobacteriosis | Microscopy of a specimen from stool or normally sterile body fluids or tissue from a site other than lungs, skin, or cervical or hilar lymph nodes that shows acid-fast bacilli of a species not identified by culture. |

Diseases	Presumptive Criteria
Kaposi's sarcoma	A characteristic gross appearance of an erythematous or violaceous plaque-like lesion or on skin or mucous membrane. (Note: Presumptive diagnosis of Kaposi's sarcoma should not be made by clinicians who have seen few cases of it.)
Pneumocystis carinii pneumonia	a. A history of dyspnea on exertion or non-productive pneumonia cough of recent onset (within the past 3 months); AND
	b. Chest X-ray evidence of diffuse bilateral interstitial infiltrates or evidence by gallium scan of diffuse bilateral pulmonary disease; AND
	c. Arterial blood gas analysis showing an arterial Po_2 of <70mm Hg or a low respiratory diffusing capacity (<80 percent of predicted values) or an increase in the alveolar-arterial oxygen tension gradient; AND
	d. No evidence of a bacterial pneumonia.
	Pneumonia, recurrent
	Recurrent (more than one episode in a one-year period), acute (new symptoms, signs, X ray evidence not present earlier) pneumonia diagnosed on clinical or radiologic grounds by the patient's physician.
Toxoplasmosis of brain	a. Recent onset of a focal neurologic abnormality consistent with intracranial disease or a reduced level of consciousness; AND
	b. Evidence by brain imaging (computed tomography or nuclear magnetic resonance) of a lesion having a mass effect or the radiographic appearance of which is enhanced by injection of contrast medium; AND
	c. Serum antibody to toxoplasmosis or successful response to therapy for toxoplasmosis.

Diseases	Presumptive Criteria
Tuberculosis, pulmonary	When bacteriologic confirmation is not available, other reports may be considered to be verified cases of pulmonary tuberculosis if the criteria of the Division of Tuberculosis Elimination, National Center for Prevention Services, CDC, are used. The criteria in use as of January 1, 1993, are available in MMWR 1990; 39 (No. RR-13):39-40.

Also called ACQUIRED IMMUNE DEFICIENCY SYNDROME. *See also* AIDS-RELATED COMPLEX, HUMAN IMMUNODEFICIENCY VIRUS, and PERSON WITH AIDS.

ACT UP: *See* AIDS COALITION TO UNLEASH POWER.

ACTG: *See* AIDS CLINICAL TRIALS GROUP.

active anal intercourse: *See* INSERTIVE ANAL INTERCOURSE.

activism: (1) A doctrine, practice, or behavior that emphasizes vigorous action for political ends. (2) A movement characterized by demonstrations, marches, disruptions, and iconography designed to draw attention to those afflicted by HIV and garner adequate support to end the AIDS epidemic.

acupressure: Compression of blood vessels by means of needles in surrounding tissues.

acupuncture: (1) A technique developed in China for treating pain or inducing anesthesia by passing needles into specific points of the body. The patient remains conscious throughout the procedure. (2) A branch of traditional Chinese medicine.

acute: (1) Sharp, severe, poignant. (2) Having sudden onset with a short and severe course. (3) Not chronic.

acute encephalopathy: (1) Any degenerative disease of the brain with a short or relatively severe course. (2) Any reversible deterioration of mental status or cognitive function.

acute HIV exanthem: A severe skin eruption or rash which manifests itself with the HUMAN IMMUNODEFICIENCY VIRUS. *Also called* EXANTHEMA.

acyclovir: (1) A drug used to treat herpes virus and sometimes used as an adjunct to *AZT*. (2) An antiviral drug which is effective against herpes simplex virus infections including types 1 and 2, varicella-zoster virus, cytomegalovirus, and Epstein-Barr virus. It is used for infections of the genitals and herpes infections of the skin. The trade name is Zovirax.

ADC: *See* AIDS DEMENTIA COMPLEX.

addiction disorder: A pathological condition involving physical and/or psychological dependence on a substance or behavior. Addiction disorders commonly involve alcohol, drugs, or engaging in sexual activities.

addictive behavior: Compulsive action motivated by physical and/ or psychological dependence on a substance or behavior. Addictive behavior often is not rational and may be self-destructive. *See also* ADDICTION DISORDER.

Addison's disease: A disease resulting from a deficiency or absence of secretion of adrenocortical hormones. This may be due to tuberculosis-induced or autoimmune-induced disease of the adrenal glands. It is characterized by anorexia, fever, tumor, hemorrhagic necrosis, weight loss, hypotension, weakness, and occasionally a discoloration of the skin. If not treated, it is usually fatal. *See also* ADRENAL INSUFFICIENCY.

adenine arabinoside: *See* VIDARABINE.

adenopathy: Swelling or enlargement of the lymph nodes.

adenovirus: One of a group of related viruses which cause disease in the upper respiratory tract. These viruses have also appeared in latent infections in some people. Many types of adenoviruses have been isolated and assigned numbers. In addition to human adenoviruses, there are also various types found in animals.

adherence: Following medication instructions for the purpose of limiting adverse effects and maximizing efficacy.

adjuvant: (1) Something that enhances the effectiveness of medical therapy. (2) A substance, especially a drug, added to a prescription to increase or hasten the action or effect of the principal ingredient. Adjuvants may involve combined treatment modalities, either concurrent or successive. (3) In immunology, a variety of substances, including inorganic gels such as alum, aluminum hydroxide, or aluminum phosphate, that increase the antigenic response.

Administration for Children and Families (ACF): An office within the Department of Health and Human Services, ACF administers 60 programs targeting needy children and families, including Head Start and the National Child Support Enforcement System. Administration for Children and Families 370 L'Enfant Promenade, Washington, DC 20447. Web site: <http://www.acf.dhhs.gov/>.

Administration on Aging (AOA): An office within the Department of Health and Human Services, the AOA provides access to a nationwide resource directory, resources for caregivers, statistical data, and many other topics relevant to an aging population. Links to all regional offices, with complete contact information included, is available from the AOA's Web site. Administration on Aging, 330 Independence Avenue, S.W., Washington, DC 20201. Telephone: (202) 619-7501; TDD: (202) 401-7575; Fax: (202) 260-1012; Eldercare Locator: (800) 677-1116. Both e-mail and Spanish language materials are available from the Web site, <http://www.aoa.dhhs.gov/>.

adolescent: An individual during the period marked by the beginning of puberty until maturity. This period is a gradual process and varies among individuals. It is classified by the National Library of Medicine as extending from age 13-18, but other institution or disciplines define it as broadly as extending from age 11-25.

adoption: The legal process of taking a child of other parents as one's own. Adoption of "AIDS babies" has been a major consequence of the epidemic since parents often desert HIV-infected newborns, are not capable of caring for them, or die leaving them orphaned. Noninfected children of HIV-positive parents may also be neglected, deserted, or orphaned.

adrenal function: The action performed by the adrenal gland.

adrenal insufficiency: Abnormally low or decreased production of adrenal corticoid hormone by the adrenal gland. Addison's disease is the result. *See also* ADDISON'S DISEASE.

adult respiratory distress syndrome (ARDS): (1) A form of lung disease in which an abnormally large amount of fluid is present in the tissue. (2) A restrictive lung disease caused by increased permeability of the pulmonary capillaries or the alveolar epithelium. The condition often develops after severe infection, trauma, or systemic illness. It has approximately a 50 percent fatality rate.

advance directives: Documentation regarding a person's wishes concerning resuscitation and artificial life support. *See also* DO NOT RESUSCITATE ORDER, NO CODE, LIVING WILL, and DURABLE POWER OF ATTORNEY FOR HEALTH CARE.

adverse effect: In pharmacology and therapeutics, the development of undesired side effects, reactions, or toxicity caused by the administration of drugs. Onset may be fast or slow.

Advil: *See* IBUPROFEN.

aerosolized pentamidine: An anti-infective drug produced as a colloidal solution and dispensed as a mist for inhaling. It is effective as a prophylaxis against *Pneumocystis carinii* pneumonia. The trade name is NebuPent.

African swine fever: A viral disease caused by an immunologically distinct agent, and first isolated in Africa. It has also been found in Brazil, Cuba, The Dominican Republic, Haiti, and western Europe. It was considered early in the epidemic to have possibly been the causative agent of the acquired immunodeficiency syndrome.

African traditional medicine: System of traditional healing based on the beliefs and practices of African peoples. Includes healing through the use of herbals, and especially the intervention of witch doctors or sorcerers. A majority of African traditional healers are women, operating within a male-dominant society. Cultural taboos forbid the discussion of safe sexual practices, which effectively blocks efforts toward prevention of HIV infection in many areas of the continent, particularly sub-Saharan Africa.

AG-1343: *See* NELFINAVIR.

Agency for Health Care Policy and Research (AHCPR): Through the Department of Health and Human Services, Public Health Service, AHCPR was established in 1989 as the lead agency responsible for supporting research designed to improve health quality, reduce health care costs, and broaden access to essential health care services. Clinical Practice Guidelines have been developed under the aegis of AHCPR. Agency for Health Care Policy and Research Office of Health Care

Information, Suite 501, Executive Office Center, 2101 East Jefferson Street, Rockville MD 20852. Telephone: (800) 358-9295. Both e-mail and Spanish language materials are available directly from the Web site, <http://www.ahcpr.gov/>.

agent: Something which causes a biological, chemical, or physical effect. Bacteria which cause a disease are agents of that disease; medicine administered to cure a disease or an illness is a therapeutic agent.

AHA: *See* AMERICAN HOSPITAL ASSOCIATION.

AHCPR: *See* AGENCY FOR HEALTH CARE POLICY AND RESEARCH.

AHG: *See* FACTOR VIII.

AHMA: *See* AMERICAN HOLISTIC MEDICAL ASSOCIATION.

AIDS: *See* ACQUIRED IMMUNODEFICIENCY SYNDROME.

AIDS Action Council: Founded in 1982, this organization functions as a representative of AIDS service facilties in Washington, DC. It lobbies Congress on AIDS-related issues, monitors federally funded research, produces various publications, and maintains a speakers' bureau. AIDS Action Council, 2033 M Street N.W., Suite 801, Washington, DC 20036. Telephone: (202) 293-2886.

AIDS Clinical Trials Group (ACTG): The National Institute of Allergy and Infectious Diseases (NIAID) trial network for AIDS drugs. NIAID contracts with institutions to perform the actual drug trials through a grant process, with a principal investigator controlling the trial. Operations Center, AIDS Clinical Trials Group, National Institutes of Health, 6101 Executive Boulevard, Suite 350, Rockville, MD 20852. Telephone: (301) 230-3150; Fax: (301) 816-0938.

AIDS Coalition to Unleash Power (ACT UP): An AIDS activist organization founded in 1987 by Larry Kramer. It was originally formed to fight for the early release of drugs that could be used in the treatment of AIDS, and is devoted to increasing public awareness of the epidemic. The organization's motto is "united in anger and committed to direct action to end the AIDS crisis." AIDS Coalition to Unleash Power 332 Bleecker St., Suite G5, New York, NY 10014. Voice mail/Fax: (212) 966-4873; e-mail: actupny@ panix.com.

AIDS dementia complex (ADC): (1) A condition in which the human immunodeficiency virus affects the brain. It can result in a loss of mental capacity. (2) A constellation of neurologic symptoms caused by infection with the human immunodeficiency virus, and characterized by global impairment of intellectual function. It is usually progressive, and interferes with normal social and occupational activities. *Also called* HIV ENCEPHALITIS, HIV ENCEPHALOPATHY, MULTIFOCAL GIANT-CELL ENCEPHALITIS, and SUBACUTE ENCEPHALITIS.

AIDS enteropathy: Any intestinal disease manifesting with the acquired immunodeficiency syndrome. *See also* ACQUIRED IMMUNO-DEFICIENCY SYNDROME.

AIDS group homes: Place where HIV-infected patients can live cheaply and safely, with support from one another, volunteers, and caregivers.

AIDS Health Service Program: A program created and implemented by the Robert Wood Johnson Foundation to assist with the high cost of AIDS. The Program accomplishes this by addressing the ways in which health care services are organized. It is funded through grants from private foundations and covers Florida, Georgia, Louisiana, New Jersey, Texas, and Washington. *See also* AIDS SERVICE DEMONSTRATION PROGRAM, AIDS-SPECIFIC MEDICAID HOME AND COMMUNITY-BASED WAIVER, and DESIGNATED AIDS CENTER PROGRAM. AIDS Health Service Program, c/o Robert Wood Johnson Foundation, P.O. Box 2316, Princeton, NJ 08540-2316. Telephone: (609) 452-8701; e-mail: mail@rwjf.org.

AIDS Knowledge Base: A textbook that covers all aspects of AIDS, prepared by health care professionals associated with the San Francisco General Hospital, the University of California, and various affiliated institutions. The print version is published by Lippincott Williams & Wilkins. It is also available electronically via HIV Insite's Web site, <http://hivinsite.ucsf.edu/>.

AIDS Medical Foundation (AMF): A nonprofit organization founded in 1982 by Dr. Mathilde Krim that promoted AIDS research and provided funding for its support. The Foundation merged with the National AIDS Research Foundation to form the

American Foundation for AIDS Research in 1985. *See also* AMERI-
CAN FOUNDATION FOR AIDS RESEARCH.

AIDS prodrome: Any sign or symptom indicative of the onset of
the acquired immunodeficiency syndrome. *See also* ACQUIRED IM-
MUNODEFICIENCY SYNDROME.

AIDS Project Los Angeles: One of the early AIDS service organizations founded in the United States. It continues to be the main service
provider in the Los Angeles area. AIDS Project Los Angeles, 1313 N.
Vine St., Los Angeles, CA 90028. Telephone: (213) 993-1600; Fax:
(213) 993-1598; California HIV/AIDS Hotline: (800) 367-AIDS;
AIDS Project Los Angeles Clientline: (213) 465-4162.

AIDS Service Demonstration Program: A program created and
implemented by the Health Resources and Services Administration
to assist with the high cost of AIDS. The Program accomplished
this by addressing the ways in which health care services are organized. It was funded by federal grants and covered Arizona, Florida,
Georgia, Illinois, Louisiana, Massachusetts, New Jersey, New York,
Pennsylvania, Puerto Rico, Texas, and Washington. The Program
preceded those funded by the Ryan White CARE Act and is no
longer in existence. *See also* AIDS HEALTH SERVICE PROGRAM, AIDS-
SPECIFIC MEDICAID HOME AND COMMUNITY-BASED WAIVERS, DESIG-
NATED AIDS CENTER PROGRAM, and RYAN WHITE CARE ACT.

AIDS service organization (ASO): An institution or consolidated
group operating at the local, state, or national level that provides
beneficial activities to individuals infected with the human immunodeficiency virus such as medical services, counseling services,
legal assistance, housing assistance, or the operation of a food bank.

AIDS Task Force for the American College Health Association:
This organization attempts to educate college students as to the reality and dangers of AIDS. HIV Disease Advisory Group for the
American College Health Association, Richard P. Keeling, MD, Director, University Health Services and Professor of Medicine, University of Wisconsin-Madison, 1552 University Ave., Madison, WI
53705. Telephone: (608) 262-1885; Fax: (608) 262-4701; e-mail:
rkeeling@facstaff.wisc.edu. *See also* AMERICAN COLLEGE HEALTH AS-
SOCIATION.

AIDS Treatment Evaluation Units (ATEU): A network of drug testing sites created by the National Institute of Allergy and Infectious Diseases (NIAID) in 1986. National Institute of Allergy and Infectious Diseases, NIAID Office of Communications, 9000 Rockville Pike, Bldg. 31, Room 7A32, Bethesda, MD 20892. Telephone: (301) 496-5717; Fax: (301) 402-0120.

AIDS Treatment Registry (ATR): A directory of New York clinical trials created in 1988 by members of the AIDS Coalition to Unleash Power (ACT-UP). The Registry was designed to provide detailed information about trials for those individuals who might want to participate. ATR is now defunct.

AIDS Vaccine Evaluation Group (AVEG): A network sponsored by the National Institute of Allergies and Infectious Disease to conduct trials of experimental vaccines meant to protect humans against HIV.

AIDSLINE: A National Library of Medicine (NLM) database that contains citations to AIDS-related literature. The citations are gleaned from various NLM databases, including CANCERLIT, HEALTH PLANNING AND ADMINISTRATION, and MEDLINE. AIDSLINE is available from the National Library of Medicine, MEDLARS Management Section, 8600 Rockville Pike, Bethesda, MD 20894. Telephone: (888) FIND-NLM. It is accessible free of charge via the World Wide Web using Internet Grateful Med's Web site, <http://igm.nlm.nih.gov>.

AIDS.NET: An electronic bulletin board that serves the deaf and hard-of-hearing communities. AIDS.NET, International Deaf/Tek, Inc., Deaftek.USA, P.O. Box 2431, Framingham, MA 01701-0404. Telephone: (508) 620-1777.

AIDSpeak: A vernacular created by public health officials, gay politicians, and AIDS activists. It has been used to describe various issues related to the disease. The jargon is bound by the usage of nonjudgmental language (e.g., "promiscuity" becomes "sexually active"), and was quickly adopted as the political tongue.

AIDSphobia: A phrase coined to denote an unrealistic fear and dread of the acquired immunodeficiency syndrome.

AIDS-related complex (ARC): A group of signs and symptoms such as fever, persistent generalized lymphadenopathy (PGL), and weight loss accompanied by the presence of human immunodeficiency virus antibodies. The immune system has already been compromised and the T-cell count is decreased. It may be a precursor to the acquired immunodeficiency syndrome. *See also* PERSON WITH AIDS-RELATED COMPLEX.

AIDS-related lymphoma: Lymphoma is a type of cancer, or malignancy, in which cancer cells are found in the lymph system. Lymphoma is divided into two broad categories, *Hodgkin's disease* and non-Hodgkin's lymphoma (NHL), based on how the diseased cells look when they are magnified.

AIDS-related virus (ARV): A virus isolated from homosexual men in 1984 in Atlanta, Georgia. It was initially thought to be similar to the human immunodeficiency virus.

AIDS-specific Medicaid Home and Community-Based Waivers: A program created and implemented by the Health Care Financing Administration to assist with the high cost of AIDS. It achieves this by addressing the ways in which health care services are organized. State and federal Medicaid money funds the program. It covers New Jersey and New Mexico. *See also* AIDS HEALTH SERVICES PROGRAM, AIDS SERVICE DEMONSTRATION PROGRAM, and DESIGNATED AIDS CENTER PROGRAM. AIDS-specific Home and Community-Based Waivers, c/o Health Care Financing Administration, Department of Health and Human Services, 200 Independence Avenue S.W., Washington, DC 20201. Telephone: (202) 690-6726.

AL 721: An egg-based compound developed to remove cholesterol from cell walls. It was tested in Phase I trials for the treatment of the acquired immunodeficiency syndrome. The majority of the research on AL 721 has been done outside of the United States, predominantly in Israel at the Weizmann Institute of Science where it was developed in 1979.

alanine: A naturally occurring, nonessential amino acid. It is an important source of energy for muscle tissue, the brain, and the central nervous system. Alanine helps in the metabolism of sugars and organic acids.

albendazole: An alternative therapy believed to be effective against microsporidiosis. It has only been approved for compassionate use treatment in the United States.

alfalfa: A leguminous plant widely grown for hay and forage. In herbal remedies, it is used to treat allergies, arthritis, morning sickness, peptic ulcers, stomach ailments, and bad breath. It is believed to cleanse the kidneys and remove toxins from the body, neutralize acids, act as a blood purifier and thinner, improve the appetite, and aid in the assimilation of protein, calcium, and other nutrients.

allergic dermatitis: *See* ATOPIC DERMATITIS.

allergic eczema: *See* ATOPIC DERMATITIS.

allergic reaction: *See* ADVERSE EFFECT.

allergy: (1) Exaggerated or abnormal reaction to substances, situations, or physical states harmless to most people. (2) An acquired hypersensitivity to a substance that does not normally cause a reaction. Essentially, it is a disorder of the immune system resulting in an antibody-antigen reaction, but in some cases the antibody cannot be demonstrated. Reaction may be immediate, or it may require repeated exposure to produce sufficient antibodies to provoke a reaction. Parts of the body most commonly displaying the results of an allergic reaction include the skin and respiratory tract.

aloe: Medicinal plant ingested by some HIV-infected patients in hopes of promoting either antiretroviral or immune system activity. Clinical studies to date are inconclusive with regard to aloe's efficacy in either case.

alopecia: Absence or loss of hair where it is normally present, especially of the head; baldness.

alpha interferon: A drug effective in preventing replication of the human immunodeficiency virus in the laboratory (in vitro). A significant limitation of its use in the living body (in vivo) is the toxic effect the drug has on humans.

alpha lipoic acid: An antioxidant that is effective in both watery and fat environments. It is believed to be effective in treating diabetic neuropathy and high liver enzyme levels.

alpha-tocopherol: *See* VITAMIN E.

alprazolam: An antianxiety drug with sedative-hypnotic actions that is effective in the treatment of panic disorder, with or without agoraphobia, and in generalized anxiety disorder. The trade name is Xanax.

altered mental state: A difference in the functional status of the mind as judged by an individual's behavior, appearance, responsiveness to stimuli of all kinds, speech, memory, and judgment.

alternative medicine: Approaches to medical diagnosis and therapy, the effectiveness of which has not been validated through the use of accepted Western methods, particularly a clinical trial process that includes a randomized, double-blind study.

alveoli: Plural of alveolus.

alveolar proteinosis: *See* PULMONARY ALVEOLAR PROTEINOSIS.

alveolus: (1) A general term used to denote a small, saclike cavity. (2) An air cell of the lung. (3) An erosion or ulcer of the gastric mucous membrane. (4) The socket of a tooth.

AMA: *See* AMERICAN MEDICAL ASSOCIATION.

ambulatory care: (1) Outpatient care, as opposed to inpatient care. (2) Treatment provided to mobile patients.

Amcil: *See* AMPICILLIN.

ameba: (1) A one-celled, microscopic organism that may infect humans, causing amebiasis. (2) A tiny, one-celled, protozoan organism that inhabits soil and water. It sends out fingerlike projections of protoplasm (pseudopodia) that enables it to move about, and through which it obtains nourishment. The pseudopodia also keep the shape of the ameba in constant flux. Ameba reproduce by binary fission, with the nucleus dividing by mitosis. Some species are parasitic in humans.

amebae: Plural of ameba.

amebiasis: The state of being infected with amebae, especially *Entamoeba histolytica*. Many patients remain asymptomatic. Those who do manifest symptoms generally present with dysentery accompanied by diarrhea, nausea, vomiting, and weakness.

amebic dysentery: Infection with *Entamoeba histolytica. See also* AMEBIASIS.

amenorrhea: absence or suppression of menstruation.

America Responds to AIDS: An AIDS education campaign launched in 1988 by the Centers for Disease Control and Prevention (as listed under C) to promote public awareness.

American Association of Blood Banks: A cooperative organization consisting of administrators, blood banks, nurses, physicians, transfusion services, and others interested in blood banking. It operates a clearinghouse for blood and blood products. The Association also conducts educational programs, trains and certifies blood bank personnel, sponsors workshops, and maintains a file on rare donors. It inspects and accredits blood banks as well. Founded in 1947, it is located at 8101 Glenbrook Rd., Bethesda, MD 20814. Telephone: (301) 907-6977; Fax: (301) 907-6895; e-mail: aabb@aabb.org.

American Association of Kidney Patients: An organization made up of persons on hemodialysis, on peritoneal dialysis, with kidney transplants, their friends and families, and professionals in the field. The Association was established in 1969, and works to educate the public about kidney disease, to fight for quality of health care, and to promote kidney donations. American Association of Kidney Patients, 1 Davis Boulevard, Suite LL7, Tampa, FL 33606. Telephone: (813) 251-0725.

American Association of Physicians for Human Rights (AAPHR): An organization made up of physicians and medical students who seek to eliminate discrimination based on affectual or sexual orientation in the health professions. The Association educates the public about homosexual health care needs, and promotes unprejudiced care for gay and lesbian clients. Founded in 1979, it is located at 2940 16th Street, Suite 105, San Francisco, CA 94103. Telephone: (415) 255-4547.

American Cancer Society (ACS): An organization made up of volunteers who support research and education in cancer detection, diagnosis, prevention, and treatment. Special services are provided to cancer patients. Founded in 1913, it is located at 1599 Clifton Road N.E., Atlanta, GA 30329-4251. Telephone: (404) 320-3333; or toll-free (800) ACS-2345.

American Civil Liberties Union (ACLU): An association which fights for the rights of people established in the Bill of Rights of the United States Constitution by providing advocacy, education, and litigation. Established in 1920, it is located at 132 W. 43rd Street, New York, NY 10036. Telephone: (212) 944-9800.

American College Health Association (ACHA): An organization consisting of institutions and individuals that is concerned with the promotion of health to college students and members of the college community. The Association provides continuing education and seminars for health professionals. Founded in 1920, it is located at P.O. Box 28937, Baltimore, MD 21240-8937. Telephone: (410) 859-1500; Fax: (410) 859-1510; e-mail: acha@access.digex.net. *See also* AIDS TASK FORCE FOR THE AMERICAN COLLEGE HEALTH ASSOCIATION.

American Foundation for AIDS Research (AmFAR): An organization dedicated to promoting AIDS research and providing funding for its support. It was founded in 1985 by the merger of the AIDS Medical Foundation and the National AIDS Research Foundation, and is headquartered at 120 Wall St., 13th floor, New York, NY 10005. Telephone: (212) 806-1600; Fax: (212) 806-1601.

American Holistic Medical Association (AHMA): Founded in 1978, it comprises licensed medical doctors, doctors of osteopathy, and medical or osteopathic students who are interested in promoting holistic health care (the integration of emotional, mental, physical, and spiritual concerns with the environment). The Association provides referrals to the public, maintains various committees, and produces several publications. American Holistic Medical Association, 6728 Old McLean Village Dr., McLean, VA 22101-3906. Telephone: (703) 556-9728; Fax: (703) 556-8729; e-mail: HolistMed@aol. com.

American Hospital Association (AHA): Founded in 1898, this organization comprises health care institutions and individuals concerned with the provision of health services. It conducts research on various aspects of the provision of health care and provides educational programs for health care personnel. American Hospital Association, One North Franklin, Chicago, IL 60606. Telephone: (312) 422-3000; Fax: (312) 422-4796.

American Medical Association (AMA): An organization made up of physicians and county medical societies. Founded in 1847 to disseminate information to its members and the public at large, the Association assists in establishing standards for continuing education, hospitals, medical schools, and residency programs. It lobbies Congress on behalf of its members concerning issues affecting the delivery of health care. The AMA also operates a library and produces various publications. American Medical Association, 515 N. State Street, Chicago, IL 60610. Telephone: (312) 464-5000.

American Public Health Association (APHA): A professional organization consisting of health care professionals and interested consumers. Founded in 1872 to seek to ensure the promotion and protection of environmental, mental, and physical health, the Association produces various publications, and is located at 1015 15th Street N.W., Washington, DC 20005-2605. Telephone: (202) 789-5600; Fax: (202) 789-5661; e-mail: comments@apha.org.

American Red Cross: Founded in 1881, this organization provides services to members of the armed forces, veterans, and their families. It also assists in disasters, and aids other Red Cross societies. This organization also operates regional blood centers, trains volunteers, and provides community services, as well as providing HIV/AIDS education programs. The Red Cross publishes service-related materials. American Red Cross offices exist throughout the United States; the main office is located at American Red Cross, Attn: Public Inquiry Office, 6th floor, 8111 Gatehouse Rd., Falls Church, VA 22042. Telephone: (703) 206-7090; e-mail: info@usa.redcross.org.

Americans for a Sound AIDS Policy (ASAP): Founded in 1987, this organization advocates a compassionate, enlightened, ethical public policy on HIV and AIDS. It seeks to educate the community in order to stop the spread of HIV, promotes early detection of infection, operates a speakers' bureau, houses an on-site collection of newspaper articles, disseminates information, and testifies to government agencies concerning AIDS-related issues. Americans for a Sound AIDS Policy, P.O. Box 17433, Washington, DC 20041. Telephone: (703) 471-7350; Fax: (703) 471-8409.

AMF: *See* AIDS MEDICAL FOUNDATION.

AmFAR: *See* AMERICAN FOUNDATION FOR AIDS RESEARCH.

amino acid: (1) Any of a large group of organic acids that link together to form the proteins necessary for life. (2) One of a large group of organic compounds containing both an amino group and a carboxyl group. They have the ability to act as both an acid and a base, and exhibit properties associated with both the amino and carboxyl groups. They serve as the building blocks for the construction of proteins, and are the end result of protein hydrolysis or digestion. Approximately 80 amino acids have been isolated in nature, with 20 being essential for human growth and metabolism.

amino acid therapy: A questionable form of AIDS therapy available outside of the United States, especially in Mexico. Beneficial results, when observed, have not been proven to be long term.

amitriptyline: A tricyclic antidepressant. It prevents the reuptake of norepinephrine and serotonin at nerve terminals and is used particularly in the treatment of endogenous depression. The trade name is Elavil.

amniocentesis: Test performed during the prenatal period to determine whether the fetus has specific, currently identifiable genetic or biochemical abnormalities. In some cases, especially in the case of maternal-fetal blood incompatibility, treatment of the fetus can occur. The procedure involves withdrawal of a sample of amniotic fluid through an ultrasound-guided syringe.

amniotic fluid: The transparent, almost colorless liquid contained in the inner membranae (amnion) which holds the suspended fetus. This liquid protects the fetus from physical impact, insulates against temperature variations, and prevents the fetus from adhering to the amnion or the amnion to the fetus. The amniotic fluid is continually absorbed and replenished.

amoxicillin: (1) A semisynthetic penicillin. (2) A semisynthetic derivative of ampicillin. It is effective against a broad spectrum of gram-positive and gram-negative bacteria, and is administered orally. Trade names include Amoxil, Polymox, Robamox, and Trimox.

Amoxil: *See* AMOXICILLIN.

amphotericin B: (1) An antibiotic agent used in the treatment of severe fungal infections. (2) An antifungal antibiotic derived from a strain of *Streptomyces nodosus*. It is administered parenterally (brought into the body by any means other than the digestive tract, such as an intravenous injection) in the treatment of such deep-seated mycotic infections as systemic candidiasis, aspergillosis, cryptococcosis, and histoplasmosis. The drug may also be applied to the skin topically in the treatment of candidiasis and related infections. The trade name is Abelcet.

ampicillin: A semi-synthetic penicillin which appears as a white, crystalline powder. When administered orally, this antibiotic is effective against various gram-negative and gram-positive bacteria. Predominantly used in the treatment of urinary system and urinary tract infections, it is also used to treat prolonged bronchial infections. Trade names include Amcil, Omnipen, Polycillin, and Principen.

Ampligen: An interferon inducing drug developed by DuPont which has received limited testing for the treatment of the acquired immunodeficiency syndrome.

amyl nitrite inhalant: A highly flammable and volatile clear liquid that causes blood vessels to relax (or dilate) when inhaled. True amyl nitrite generally requires a prescription, unlike butyl nitrite. It is used recreationally. *Also called* RUSH and POPPERS.

amyloidosis: A metabolic disorder characterized by a starchlike protein-polysaccharide known as "amyloid" being deposited in organs and tissues. It is believed to be the result of dysfunctioning of the reticuloendothelial system and abnormal immunoglobulin synthesis. There is no known method of preventing formation of amyloid deposits other than controlling the primary disease with which it is associated.

anabolic steroids: Testosterone, or a hormone similar to it, that when ingested, stimulates cell growth. Both male and female athletes sometimes use anabolic steroids to "bulk up" for sports and games. These substances, while illegal for competitive athletes to use, have been proven helpful for men suffering from HIV wasting. The advantage is that anabolic steroids increase lean body mass rather than fat tissue, leading to gains in strength. Preliminary studies indicate that resistance training combined with moderate doses of an anabolic steroid increase strength faster than ingestion of the drug alone.

ANAC: *See* ASSOCIATION OF NURSES IN AIDS CARE.

Anafranil: *See* CLOMIPRAMINE.

anal digital intercourse: Sexual intercourse by insertion of a finger into the anus.

anal intercourse: Sexual intercourse by insertion of the penis into the anus. *Also called* ANAL SEX. *See also* INSERTIVE ANAL INTERCOURSE and RECEPTIVE ANAL INTERCOURSE.

anal manual intercourse: Sexual intercourse by insertion of a hand into the anus.

anal sex: *See* ANAL INTERCOURSE.

anal squamous-cell carcinoma: A form of carcinoma located on the anus that develops from the flat, scaly, epithelial cells of the epidermis (those cells that form the outer surface of the body, and line the internal surfaces).

anal wart: (1) A small tumorous growth, caused by a virus, located on the anus. (2) A circumscribed cutaneous lesion located on the anus. It is caused by a human papillomavirus, and is transmitted by contact.

analgesic: (1) Relieving pain. (2) An agent which alleviates pain.

anatomy: (1) The structure of an organism. (2) The branch of science dealing with the structure of organisms.

Ancobon: *See* FLUCYTOSINE.

anemia: (1) A condition in which there is a reduction in the number or volume of red blood cells. (2) A sign of various diseases characterized by a reduction in the number of erythrocytes (circulating red blood cells) per cubic millimeter in the quantity of hemoglobin per 100 milliliters, or in the volume of packed red cells per 100 milliliters of blood. The balance between blood loss and blood production is disturbed, and the content of hemoglobin necessary to carry oxygen throughout the body is decreased.

anergy: A reduced response to several specific antigens.

anger: (1) A strong feeling of displeasure. (2) A feeling of displeasure or exasperation in response to a person, action, situation, or object. This emotion generally results in the desire to retaliate against whatever supposedly spawned it. Anger (under various circumstances) has been credited as being necessary for survival as it assists in mobilizing a response to adverse situations.

angular cheilitis: *See* PERLÈCHE.

angular cheilosis: *See* PERLÈCHE.

angular stomatitis: *See* PERLÈCHE.

anilinctus: *See* ANILINGUS.

anilingus: Sexual activity in which the mouth and tongue are used to stimulate the anus. *Also called* ANILINCTUS and RIMMING.

anorectal disease: A pathological condition of the anus and rectum, or the area joining the two, which is manifested by a characteristic set of clinical signs and symptoms.

anorexia: The lack or loss of appetite for food. This is common in the onset of fevers and systemic illnesses, psychiatric illnesses, depression, malaise, and in pathological conditions of the alimentary tract, especially the stomach.

anoxia: Without oxygen.

Ansamycin: *See* RIFABUTIN.

anthrax: An acute, bacterial, infectious disease caused by *Bacillus anthracis*. It generally attacks cattle, goats, horses, or sheep, but may be passed on to humans through contact with infected animals, their discharges, or contaminated animal products. Failure to properly treat anthrax may be fatal. *Also called* CHARBON, MILZBRAND, and SPLENIC FEVER.

anthropology: The branch of science dealing with man, especially his origin, development, and culture. Major divisions include physical anthropology, cultural anthropology, linguistics, and archaeology.

anthroposophy: A twentieth century religious movement growing out of theosophy and centering on human development.

antibacterial: (1) Destroying or suppressing the growth or reproduction of bacteria. (2) A substance that destroys or suppresses the growth or reproduction of bacteria.

antibody: (1) A specialized protein substance produced by certain lymphocytes in response to the presence of an antigen to form the basis for immunity. (2) A protein substance, comprised of immunoglobulin molecules with a specific amino acid sequence, developed in response to the presence of an antigen. The antibody interacts only with the antigen which caused its creation, or with those that are closely related. This relationship between antigen and antibody forms the basis for humoral immunity. The presence of antibodies may be linked to vaccination, previous infection, perinatal transfer of bodily fluids between mother and fetus, or accidentally through unknown exposure. The body also possesses natural antibodies which react without apparent contact with the specific antigen.

antibody testing: The procedure used to determine the presence of an antibody. *See also* ANTIBODY.

anticonvulsant: (1) Any agent that prevents or relieves convulsions. (2) Preventing or relieving convulsions.

antidepressant: An agent that prevents, cures, relieves, or alleviates depression. *See also* DEPRESSION.

antidiuretic hormone: *See* VASOPRESSIN.

antifungal: Any agent that kills fungi, inhibits the growth or reproduction of fungi, or is used to treat fungal infections.

antigen: Any substance which, under specific conditions, has the ability to induce a particular immune response and to react with the product of that response. The antigen induces the synthesis of an antibody; it is this interaction which forms the basis for immunity.

antihemophilic factor A: *See* FACTOR VIII.

antihemophilic globulin: *See* FACTOR VIII.

antimoniotungstate: (1) A drug found to be poisonous to the blood when tested for treating infection with the human immunodeficiency virus. (2) This drug was developed in the 1970s as a potential treatment for Creutzfeldt-Jakob disease. It inhibits the reverse transcriptase, and has been tested in Phase I and II trials for treatment of infection with the human immunodeficiency virus. It has consistently exhibited hematologic toxicity in these tests. *Also called* HPA-23.

antimycobacterial: (1) Effective against mycobacteria. (2) An agent that is effective against mycobacteria. *See also* MYCOBACTERIAL INFECTION.

antineoplastic: (1) An agent that prevents the development, growth, or spread of malignant cells. (2) Preventing the development, growth, or spread of malignant cells.

antioxidant: Any agent that prevents or inhibits oxidation.

antiretroviral: Any agent that destroys a retrovirus or inhibits its replication.

antiviral: Any substance that destroys a virus or inhibits its replication.

antiviral drug therapy: The administration of an agent that destroys a virus or inhibits its replication.

anus: The terminal orifice of the digestive tract, which serves as an outlet for the rectum, located in the fold between the buttocks.

anxiety: (1) A feeling of apprehension, worry, uneasiness, or dread. (2) Painful uneasiness of mind, usually over an anticipated ill or the future. (3) Abnormal apprehension and fear often accompanied by physiological signs, such as sweating and increased pulse rate, by doubt about the nature of the threat itself, and by self-doubt.

anxiety disorder: Name for an entire group of neurotic conditions that may include anxiety, panic disorder, obsessive-compulsive disorder, post-traumatic stress syndrome, and others. The *Diagnostic and Statistical Manual,* Fourth Edition, contains a full discussion of these disorders, as well as generalized anxiety disorder.

AOA: *See* ADMINISTRATION ON AGING.

APHA: *See* AMERICAN PUBLIC HEALTH ASSOCIATION.

aphtha: A small ulcer on a mucous membrane of the mouth.

aphthae: Plural of aphtha.

aphthous: Pertaining to, or characterized by, aphthae.

aphthous stomatitis: Small oral ulcer caused by prolonged or recurrent inflammation of tissues in the mouth. Sometimes called canker sore. Cause is thought to be linked to the immune system, which can be compromised due to disease, emotional stress, fever, or even foods to which a susceptible individual is sensitive. *Also called* APHTHOUS ULCER.

aphthous ulcer: *See* APHTHOUS STOMATITIS.

apnea: (1) Cessation of breathing. (2) Asphyxia.

apoplexy: *See* CEREBROVASCULAR ACCIDENT.

ara-A: *See* VIDARABINE.

ARC: *See* AIDS-RELATED COMPLEX.

ARDS: *See* ADULT RESPIRATORY DISTRESS SYNDROME.

arenavirus: (1) A group of RNA viruses that cause a variety of diseases in humans. (2) Any of a group of viruses consisting of multishaped virions that have 4 large and 1-3 small segments of single-stranded RNA. The presence of ribosomes gives the virions a sandy appearance. The principal virus in this group is the lymphocytic choriomeningitis virus (LCM virus). Also included are the American hemorrhagic fever viruses and the Lassa fever virus. Rodents typically serve as hosts for the viruses.

arginine: An amino acid.

aroma therapy: Use of scent to alleviate stress or other maladies.

art therapy: Use of expression through some artistic means (e.g., sculpture, drawing, or painting) to ameliorate either a physical or emotional condition. In the HIV/AIDS arena, art therapy has been used most effectively as a coping tool among HIV-positive and AIDS patients of all ages and genders. It is also used as a tool for prevention, particularly among adolescents and adults in high-risk categories.

arthralgia: Pain in a joint.

artificial insemination: The mechanical injection of semen, which is capable of fertilization, into the vagina.

ARV: *See* AIDS-RELATED VIRUS.

ASAP: *See* AMERICANS FOR A SOUND AIDS POLICY.

Ascomycetes: (1) The sac fungi. (2) The largest class of Eumycetes, the true fungi. They are characterized by a sac that encloses the spores. Included in this group are yeasts, mildews, blue molds, and truffles.

ascorbic acid: (1) Vitamin C. (2) A water-soluble vitamin found in many fruits and vegetables. Ascorbic acid is required for proper functioning of many enzymes.

aseptic meningitis: The common name for a mild form of meningitis. Most cases are caused by viruses. *See also* MENINGITIS.

ASO: *See* AIDS SERVICE ORGANIZATION.

asparagine: A nonessential amino acid.

aspartic acid: A nonessential amino acid occurring in proteins.

aspergillomycosis: *See* ASPERGILLOSIS.

aspergillosis: (1) A fungal infection. (2) Infection caused by *Aspergillus* and characterized by granulomatous lesions in the tissues or on any mucous surface. Areas commonly affected include the skin, lungs, aural canal, nasal sinuses, urethra, and occasionally in the bones or meninges. *Also called* ASPERGILLOMYCOSIS.

Aspergillus: A genus of fungi in the family Moniliaceae. After sexual development, it is classed with the Ascomycetes. This genus includes several species of molds, some of which are opportunistic pathogens.

aspirin: (1) Acetylsalicylic acid. (2) A drug having anti-inflammatory, analgesic, and antipyretic effects. Used for relief of pain and fever, for treatment of rheumatoid arthritis and osteoarthritis, and for antiplatelet therapy.

assisted living services: (1) Generally, a housing arrangement that includes private or semiprivate quarters for residents, with at least some meals prepared and eaten communally and cleaning and laundry services available. AIDS patients who are either homeless or unable to care for themselves may live in an assisted living community with other such patients. (2) May also refer to patients who stay within their own homes and acquire help with activities of daily living, particularly meals, cleaning, and personal care.

assisted suicide: Taking one's own life with help from another person. Assistance may include acquisition and delivery of drugs, a weapon, or other means of self-destruction.

Association of Nurses in AIDS Care (ANAC): Founded in 1987, this organization consists of nurses and health care professionals involved in the care of persons with AIDS. It serves as a network for its members, provides support services, promotes public awareness and education regarding AIDS issues, and advocates for the rights of those infected with the human immunodeficiency virus. Association of Nurses in AIDS Care, 11250 Roger Bacon Dr., Suite 8, Reston, VA 20190-5202. Telephone: (703) 925-0081 or toll-free (800) 260-6780; Fax: (703) 435-4390, e-mail: AIDSNURSES@aol. com.

asthma: (1) A condition in which periodically recurring sudden attacks of difficulty in breathing are accompanied by coughing and wheezing. (2) A condition characterized by paroxysmal shortness of breath accompanied by wheezing caused by spasmodic contractions of the bronchi or bronchial tubes or by swelling of the bronchial mucous membrane. Asthma may coexist with other allergies, or be caused by an allergic reaction. Secondary factors influence the recurrence and severity of attacks such as physical fatigue, mental or emotional stress, or pollutant irritants.

ASTRA Pharmaceutical Products, Inc.: The Swedish-based company that owns the drug foscarnet. ASTRA Pharmaceutical Products, Inc., 50 Otis Street, P.O. Box 4500, Westborough, MA 01581-4500. Telephone: (508) 366-1100; Fax: (508)366-7406.

astragalus: A genus of leguminous plants or many species, with some being poisonous.

asymptomatic: Exhibiting or eliciting no symptoms.

ATEU: *See* AIDS TREATMENT EVALUATION UNITS.

athlete's foot: *See* TINEA PEDIS.

Ativan: *See* LORAZEPAM.

atopic dermatitis: A chronic inflammation of the skin of unknown cause, and characterized by severe itching leading to scratching or rubbing which in turn produces lesions. Individuals affected generally have a hereditary predisposition to irritable skin. *Also called* ALLERGIC DERMATITIS, ALLERGIC ECZEMA, and ATOPIC ECZEMA.

atopic diathesis: An allergic condition which makes the body tissues more susceptible to certain diseases.

atopic eczema: *See* ATOPIC DERMATITIS.

ATR: *See* AIDS TREATMENT REGISTRY.

atrophic candidiasis: Infection with a fungus of the genus *Candida* which causes atrophy. It usually involves the skin or mucous membranae. *See also* ATROPHY.

atrophy: (1) A wasting away; a decrease in size of a cell, tissue, or organ. (2) To undergo or cause atrophy.

attitude to death: State of mind in which individuals approach death, their own or someone else's. Cross-disciplinary studies indicate that multiple losses, such as have occurred within the HIV/AIDS pandemic, adversely affect not only individuals but entire communities impacted by the disease. On the other hand, a dying person's beliefs about death may affect his or her ease of passing.

attitude to health: State of mind that influences knowledge, beliefs, and behavior with regard to health status. Particularly important in preventive medicine, an individual's attitude toward health has a bearing on participation or nonparticipation in risky behaviors.

audiology: Study of hearing.

auscultation: Act of listening for sounds within the body, especially with a stethoscope. Part of physical examination.

autoimmune mechanism: (1) The response that produces antibodies against the body's own tissues. (2) The response that produces the condition in which the body recognizes itself as foreign, and forms a humoral and cellular response against the body's own tissues.

autologous transfusion: A transfusion of blood that has either been donated in advance by the patient or collected at the site of surgery during the procedure. This process is performed in order to prevent exposure to the human immunodeficiency virus and other blood-borne diseases.

autopsy: A postmortem examination of the body, including organs and tissues, in order to determine the cause of death or pathological changes. *Also called* NECROPSY or POSTMORTEM EXAMINATION.

AVEG: *See* AIDS VACCINE EVALUATION GROUP.

Aventyl: *See* NORTRIPTYLINE.

Avlosulfon: *See* DAPSONE.

ayurveda: *See* AYURVEDIC MEDICINE.

ayurvedic medicine: System of medicine originating in south Asia as part of Hindu culture and practice. The goal is to improve or maintain health by sustaining harmony between the mind and the body. Yoga, herbal compounds, and massage are all used in the practice of ayurvedic medicine.

azathioprine: An immunosuppressive agent, created from a cytotoxic chemical substance, and used for the prevention of transplant rejection in organ transplantation. Also under investigation for use in the treatment of autoimmune diseases. The trade name is Imuran.

azidothymidine: *See* ZIDOVUDINE.

azithromycin: A semi-synthetic macrolide antibiotic structurally related to erythromycin. It has been used in the treatment of *Mycobacterium avium intracellulare* infections, toxoplasmosis, and cryptosporidiosis. The trade name is Zithromax.

azotemia: An excess of nitrogenous bodies, especially urea, in the blood. *See also* UREMIA.

AZT: *See* ZIDOVUDINE.

AZT-failure: Any indication that the condition of a person taking at least 500 mg per day of azidothymidine in excess of six months is worsening.

AZT-ineligibility: Any condition which prohibits a person from taking azidothymidine (e.g., low white blood cell count, severe anemia, administration of incompatible drugs).

AZT-intolerance: Any negative, severe, side effect resulting from the administration of azidothymidine that requires discontinuation of the drug.

B cells: *See* B LYMPHOCYTE.

B lymphocyte: A type of lymphocyte that comes from the bone marrow, and is found in the blood, lymph, and connective tissue. When stimulated by an antigen, the B-cell lymphocyte proliferates and differentiates into plasma cells and memory B cells with the cooperation of helper T cells and macrophages. This clone is specific for the antigen for which it was produced.

bacillary angiomatosis: Acute infectious disease sometimes present in immunocompromised HIV-infected patients. In cases of severe immune compromise, the prognosis for recovery is poor. Signs and symptoms include skin lesions that, if infected, can destroy underlying bone. The bacteria may also proliferate and spread to organs throughout the body, especially the liver, bone marrow, spleen, and lymph nodes. The disease is sometimes treated successfully with antibiotics.

bacillary dysentery: Disorder of the intestines, usually the colon, marked by abdominal cramping and pain and diarrhea. Bacillary dysentery is caused by various *Shigella* bacteria and may lead to severe toxemia.

Bacillus anthracis: An aerobic bacteria belonging to the genus *Bacillus*. It is the causative agent of anthrax.

baclofen: A muscle relaxant that is administered orally for the treatment of spasticity in spinal disorders.

bacteremia: The presence of bacteria in the blood.

bacteria: Plural of bacterium.

bacterial infection: The state or condition in which the body or part of it is invaded by bacteria which, under certain conditions, multiply and cause injurious effects.

bacterial pneumonia: Pneumonia caused by bacteria.

bacteriology: The study of bacteria, either as a branch of medicine or as a science.

bacteriophage: A virus that infects bacteria. They are found throughout nature, and have been isolated in excrement, polluted water, and sewage.

bacterium: Any of the unicellular microorganisms of the class Schizomycetes. The organism is usually contained within a cell wall, and multiplication is by cell division (fission). They may be aerobic or anaerobic, motile or nonmotile, and may exist independently, in decaying matter, as parasites, or as pathogens. *See also* GRAM-NEGATIVE BACTERIA and GRAM-POSITIVE BACTERIA.

Bactrim: *See* TRIMETHOPRIM/SULFAMETHOXAZOLE.

BAL: *See* BRONCHOALVEOLAR LAVAGE.

Barbados leg: *See* ELEPHANTIASIS.

Baridol: *See* BARIUM SULFATE.

barium study: (1) A test used in examining the gastrointestinal tract. (2) Any test involving the use of barium sulfate as a radiopaque (prohibiting the passage of X rays and other forms of radiant energy) contrast medium for distinguishing anatomical areas in the gastrointestinal tract.

barium sulfate: (1) An opaque substance that is swallowed to assist in the examination of the stomach and intestines. (2) An odorless, tasteless, fine, white powder used as a contrast medium in roentgenography (X rays) of the gastrointestinal tract. The trade names are Barosperse, Esophotrast, and Baridol. *Also called* BLANC FIXE.

Barosperse: *See* BARIUM SULFATE.

Bartonella henselae: A species of gram-negative bacteria that is the causative agent of bacillary angiomatosis. It can also cause cat-scratch disease in AIDS patients and other immunocompromised patients.

basal cell carcinoma: A tumor of the skin that rarely metastasizes. Usually, it manifests as a small, shiny papule. The lesion grows until it appears as a whitish border surrounding a central ulcer.

baseline: A known or initial observation or value used for comparison in measuring the response to experimental intervention or stimulus (e.g., a person's T4-cell count upon entering a clinical trial).

basophil: (1) A cell or part of a cell that stains readily with basic dyes. (2) An endocrine found in the anterior lobe of the pituitary gland. It produces the substance that stimulates the adrenal cortex to secrete adrenal cortical hormone. (3) A granular leukocyte characterized by the possession of coarse, bluish-black granules of varying size that stain intensely with basic dyes.

bathhouse: A facility resembling a public bathhouse, but used primarily for anonymous sexual encounters. Generally equipped with both private and public rooms and operated for profit. Bathhouses came under heavy fire in 1983 after it was established that the human immuno-deficiency virus is transmitted through sexual intercourse.

BCG vaccine: A tuberculosis vaccine made from a freeze-dried preparation of a live strain of *Mycobacterium bovis*. Regularly used for the vaccination of children only in areas with a high incidence rate of tuberculosis in the United States. It is recommended only for immunizing high-risk persons.

bedsore: *See* DECUBITUS ULCER.

bee propolis: Resin-like substance obtained from beehives, full of substances thought to have antimicrobial or antimycotic activity when applied topically.

behavior modification: A technique employed to alter animal or human behavior through application of the principles of conditioning. Rewards and reinforcements, or punishments, are administered to establish desired habits or patterns of behavior.

beneficiary: Person or persons designated to receive proceeds from an estate upon the death of an individual.

benign: (1) Not recurrent or progressive. (2) The opposite of malignant.

benzodiazepine: Any of a group of minor tranquilizers having a common molecular structure and similar pharmacological activities. Used as sedatives, anticonvulsants, muscle relaxants, and to provide hypnotic effects.

bereavement: The state involving loss, especially from death.

beta carotene: Found in many fresh fruits and vegetables, beta carotene is a powerful antioxidant that minimizes the cellular damage caused by free radicals.

beta cell: The cell that secretes insulin and composes the bulk of the islets of Langerhans (Langerhans cell).

Beta-sitosterol: *See* B-SITOSTEROL.

beta₂-microglobulin: A small protein found in human cells that serves as one subunit of class I major histocompatibility antigens (the system that has the ability to stimulate an immune response that causes the rejection of a transplant when a donor and recipient are mismatched). With HIV infection, beta₂ protein is released into the blood as cells are destroyed by the virus. This may serve as an indicator that T4 cells are being destroyed and the immune system weakened.

Biaxin: *See* CLARITHROMYCIN.

bibliotherapy: The reading of books for treatment of mental disorders or for mental health.

bilirubin: The orange or yellowish pigment in bile. It is produced by the degradation of erythrocyte hemoglobin in reticuloendothelial cells in the bone marrow, the spleen, and elsewhere. It is chemically altered in the liver and excreted as the water-soluble pigment in the bile. If bilirubin accumulates, it may lead to jaundice.

binding site: The reactive part of a macromolecule that directly participates in its specific combination with another molecule.

biochemistry: The chemistry of living organisms and of vital processes.

bioelectromagnetic therapy: One of seven categories in a classification of alternative medicine practices developed by the National Center for Complementary and Alternative Medicine. Bioelectromagnetics is concerned with the unconventional use of electromagnetic fields for medical, especially therapeutic, purposes.

biofeedback: Part of mind-body medicine, which is one of seven categories in a classification of alternative medicine practices developed by the National Center for Complementary and Alternative Medicine. Biofeedback is a behavioral training program wherein individuals learn to control their own autonomic nervous system, thereby attaining the ability to control such bodily functions as heart rate, blood pressure, skin temperature, or muscle relaxation.

biology: The science that deals with the phenomena of life and living organisms in general.

biomaterial dumping: The sale of a natural or synthetic substance used to replace a bodily bone, tissue, etc. in a large quantity at a low price, especially in a foreign market at a price below that of the domestic market.

biopsy: The excision of tissue from a living body for microscopic examination. It is usually performed to establish a diagnosis.

biotin: Component of the vitamin B complex.

bipolar disorder: Formerly known as manic-depressive disorder, individuals afflicted with this mental illness are characterized by experiencing wide mood swings that include periods of severe depression as well as periods of mania.

bisexual: An individual exhibiting bisexuality.

bisexuality: (1) Sexual attraction to persons of both sexes. (2) Practicing both heterosexual and homosexual behavior.

blackout: (1) The sudden loss of consciousness. (2) A condition characterized by a temporary loss of consciousness and failure of vision, due to reduced blood circulation to the brain. *Also called* SYNCOPE.

blanc fixe: *See* BARIUM SULFATE.

bleach kit: Supplies used by injection drug users to clean hypodermic syringes and works.

bleomycin: (1) Any of a mixture of antibiotics produced by a strain of *Streptomyces verticillus.* (2) Any of a group of antitumor antibiotics produced by a strain of *Streptomyces verticillus.* It is used in conjunction with other chemotherapies for treatment of Hodgkin's disease and non-Hodgkin's lymphomas, squamous cell carcinomas of the head and neck, testicular carcinoma, and uterine cervix carcinoma. Fever, nausea, and vomiting are common side effects. Major side effects include occasionally fatal dose-related pneumonitis, pulmonary fibrosis, and severe skin reactions.

blood bank: Any facility where whole blood and certain components are collected, processed, typed, and stored until needed for transfusion. *See also* TISSUE BANK.

blood coagulation test: A laboratory test for evaluating an individual's clotting mechanism.

blood disease: *See* HEMATOLOGIC DISORDER.

blood glucose: Sugar in the blood; the form in which carbohydrate is carried in the blood, usually in a concentration of 70-100 mg per 100 ml. An abnormally diminished concentration of blood glucose is hypoglycemia; an abnormally increased amount in hyperglycemia.

blood products: Anything made naturally or artificially concerning the blood.

blood sedimentation: *See* ERYTHROCYTE SEDIMENTATION RATE.

blood splash: The accidental scattering of blood so as to wet or soil an individual.

blood sugar: *See* BLOOD GLUCOSE.

blood supply: The amount of blood stored and available for use.

blood test: *See* HEMATOLOGIC TEST.

blood transfusion: The replacement of blood or one of its components.

blood-brain barrier: Physical barriers found on the capillary walls of the brain that prevent the transmission of harmful substances from other parts of the body into the brain and the cerebrospinal fluid.

blow: *See* COCAINE.

Blue Cross and Blue Shield Association: Founded in 1982, the Association comprises local Blue Cross and Blue Shield Plans for health insurance in the United States, Canada, the United Kingdom, and Jamaica. It works to provide national services to local Plans, promote improvement of public health, and secure public acceptance of health insurance services. The Association produces various publications, and has an on-site library. Blue Cross and Blue Shield Association, 225 N. Michigan Ave., Chicago, IL 60611. Telephone: (312) 297-6000.

BLV: *See* BOVINE LEUKEMIA VIRUS.

bodily fluid: Any of the liquids contained in, or produced by, the human body (e.g., blood, perspiration, saliva, semen, tears, vaginal secretions).

body modification: Altering the appearance of the body through invasive means, including tattooing, piercing, or cosmetic surgery.

body piercing: *See* BODY MODIFICATION.

boil: *See* FURUNCLE.

bone marrow aspiration: Withdrawal of a sample of marrow, a soft, organic material that fills cavities in bones, for diagnostic purposes. Many blood diseases, malignancies, and infections can be diagnosed in this way.

bone marrow suppression: Any chemical or process that suppresses the production of cells or the maturation of cells within the bone marrow.

booting: The procedure practiced by IV drug users in which blood is withdrawn into the drug-filled syringe, prior to injecting the entire contents. The process is supposed to enhance the drug-induced high. Booting increases the risk for transmission of the human immunodeficiency virus by providing increased contact between blood and needle/syringe.

bootleg: To produce, carry, or sell illegally.

bovine leukemia virus: A virus found in cattle that is similar in structure to the human T-cell leukemia virus.

boycott: Refusal to patronize a business or purchase a product in order to make a political statement.

brachioproctic eroticism: Penetration of the rectum with the hand and forearm to induce sexual stimulation. Also called fisting or fist-fucking.

brain imaging: The use of X ray or nuclear techniques that produce an image representative of the brain.

brain scan: The process used to detect aberrations in the function or structure of the brain by injecting radioactive isotopes into the circulatory system.

breakthrough pain: Pain that occurs in spite of adherence to potent pain medications.

breast-feeding: The nursing of an infant at a mother's breast.

Bristol-Myers Squibb Company: A pharmaceutical company that holds the license for didanosine (ddI), and other health care products. Bristol-Myers Squibb Company, P.O. Box 9445, McLean, VA 22102-9445. Telephone: (800) 736-0003.

broad-spectrum antibiotics: Effective against a variety of microorganisms.

bronchi: Plural of bronchus.

bronchitis: Inflamation of the bronchial tubes.

bronchoalveolar lavage (BAL): The washing out of the bronchus and alveoli to remove irritants, or to diagnose inflammation or infection.

bronchoscopy: A procedure to examine the bronchi in which an instrument, a bronchoscope, is inserted orally for the purpose of taking specimens for culture and biopsy. It is used to diagnose pulmonary disorders such as *Pneumocystis carinii* pneumonia.

bronchus: (1) Any of the larger air passages of the lungs. (2) One of the large branches of the trachea.

brush biopsy: A biopsy in which tiny brushes are used to remove cells or tissue.

B-sitosterol: A natural plant steroid used as an oral agent against excess cholesterol in the blood.

budding: A method of asexual reproduction in which a budlike process grows from the side or end of the parent and develops into a new organism (the larger part is considered the parent and the smaller one the bud). The bud may remain attached, or separate and live independently of the parent. This form of reproduction is common in lower animals and plants, including many of the fungi that invade the human body.

buddy program: A program that pairs a healthy individual with one who is ill and alone. The healthy buddy is on call in the event of emergency, assists with activities of daily living, and provides companionship.

buffalo hump: Side effect of some protease inhibitors in which a layer of fat tissue gathers in the area of the cervical spine, leading to a disfiguring hump. The side effect was not reported in initial clinical trials but appears to occur following longer term use of protease inhibitors. *See also* SIDE EFFECT.

burdock: Any of several plants of the composite family, with large basal leaves and purple-flowered heads covered with hooked prickles. The root is thought to be a blood purifier and cleanser. It is also believed that the root aids in healing skin blemishes, arthritis, and rheumatism as well as promoting healthy kidney function.

Bureau of Primary Health Care: One of four bureaus of the Health Resources and Services Administration, the Bureau of Primary Health Care assures that underserved and vulnerable people get the health care they need. The Bureau's mission is to increase access to comprehensive primary and preventive health care and to improve the health status of underserved and vulnerable populations. Bureau of Primary Health Care, East West Towers, 4350 East West Highway, Bethesda, MD 20814. Telephone: (301) 594-4110.

Burkitt's lymphoma: (1) A form of cancer characterized most often by tumors in the jaw or abdominal area. (2) A form of highly undifferentiated lymphoblastic lymphoma manifested most often in the jaw or as an abdominal mass. It involves sites other than the lymph nodes and reticuloendothelial system. This form of lymphoma is rare in the United States, and is found most commonly in Central Africa. The Epstein-Barr virus has been implicated as the causative agent.

burnout: Combination of physical and emotional exhaustion, generally precipitated by prolonged period of stress. Often found in the workplace among employees who feel little control over and no joy in their work.

Busse-Buschke disease: *See* CRYPTOCOCCOSIS.

butyl nitrite inhalant: A liquid compound that dilates blood vessels and reduces blood pressure when inhaled. It is used recreationally to produce a brief high. Unlike amyl nitrite, butyl nitrite does not require a prescription. *Also called* RUSH and POPPERS.

butyrophenone: Any of a class of structurally related antipsychotic agents. The prototype is haloperidol.

buyers' club: *See* BUYERS' GROUP.

buyers' group: A group that imports from other countries drugs not yet approved for use in the United States by the Food and Drug Administration. *Also called* BUYERS' CLUB.

C

cachexia: *See* HIV WASTING SYNDROME.

caesarean section: Surgical delivery of a fetus through an incision in the mother's abdomen. *Also called* CE-SAEREAN SECTION.

caffeine: A bitter, crystalline alkaloid present in coffee, tea, kola nuts, etc. It stimulates the central nervous system, mainly affecting the cerebrum, has a diuretic effect on the kidneys, stimulates striated muscles, and has a group of effects on the cardiovascular system.

CAIDS: *See* COMMUNITY ACQUIRED IMMUNE DEFICIENCY SYNDROME.

calcium: Metallic element found in many foods and essential for strong bones and teeth and other important activities within the body.

Calcium Folinate: *See* FOLINIC ACID.

Campylobacter: (1) A genus of bacteria that is a cause of diarrhea in AIDS patients. (2) A genus of bacteria made up of gram-negative, nonspore-forming, spiral shaped, motile rods with polar flagella. These bacteria are found in both humans and animals in the intestinal tract, oral cavity, and reproductive systems. Certain species are pathogenic and may cause enteritis or systemic disease in humans, and spontaneous abortion in some animals.

CAN: *See* CURE AIDS NOW.

cancer: (1) A harmful new growth anywhere in the body. (2) A malignant tumor. Cancer cells possess the properties of invasion and metastasis, and comprise a broad group of neoplasms. These are divided into two groups: carcinoma (those originating in epithelial tissues) and sarcoma (those developing from connective tissues and structures having their origin in mesodermal tissues).

Cancer Information Service: *See* NATIONAL CANCER INSTITUTE.

Candida: (1) A fungi that is a common cause of opportunistic infections in people with AIDS. (2) A genus of yeast-like fungi which is characterized by the production of yeast cells. Reproduction is performed by budding. It is commonly part of the flora of the mouth, skin, intestinal tract, and vagina. Candida may cause a variety of infections such as candidiasis or vaginitis.

candidal endocarditis: Infection of the internal lining or structures of the heart with fungi of the genus *Candida*.

candidemia: The presence of fungi of the genus *Candida* in the blood. This condition usually results from systemic candidiasis or candidal endocarditis.

candidiasis: (1) A fungal infection which occurs in several places in the body, including the mouth or throat (thrush), vagina, and on the skin; a common opportunistic infection in people with AIDS. (2) Infection with a fungus of the genus *Candida*. It usually infects the moist cutaneous areas of the body (skin or mucous membrane), and is chiefly caused by *Candida albicans. Also called* CANDIDOSIS, OIDIOMYCOSIS, and MONILIASIS.

candidosis: *See* CANDIDIASIS.

cannabis: (1) Hemp. (2) The dried flowering tops of hemp plants which contain the euphoric properties. It is classified as a hallucinogenic and is prepared as bhang, ganja, hashish, and marijuana.

capsicum: General term that refers to the fruit of all pepper plants.

carcinoma: (1) Any of several kinds of cancerous growths made up of epithelial cells. (2) A new growth or malignant tumor made up of epithelial cells. These neoplasms tend to infiltrate the surrounding tissue and give rise to metastases. It may affect almost any part of the body or its organs.

cardiology: The study of the heart and its functions.

cardiovascular syphilis: (1) Syphilis involving the heart and great blood vessels. (2) A form of tertiary syphilis involving the heart and great blood vessels, especially the aorta. Aortic aneurysms and aortic insufficiency often result, thereby causing damage to the intima and media of the great blood vessels. Congestive heart failure may result.

caregiver: An individual charged with, or assuming, the responsibility of watching over, or attending to, a physically or mentally ill person.

carnitine: Chemical necessary for metabolizing certain acids. Sometimes used therapeutically to treat myopathy caused by a deficiency in carnitine.

cascara sagrada: Chemical derived from the dried bark of the buckthorn that is used as a laxative.

case doubling time: The amount of time necessary for the occurrence of a disease to double in number.

case history: The collection of data concerning an individual regarding his or her medical, family, psychiatric, and social history. This information is gathered to provide a better understanding of the patient, and is useful in analyzing and diagnosing the present illness.

case management: The handling of an individual incidence of disease, injury, or other medical abnormality, with the result being care and/or treatment that is satisfactory under the circumstances.

case-fatality rate: The proportion of deaths caused by the occurrence of a disease.

casual social contact: (1) The act or state of occasionally or superficially meeting or touching someone. (2) Not intimate.

CAT scan: *See* COMPUTERIZED AXIAL TOMOGRAPHIC SCAN.

cathartic: (1) Causing purgation of the bowels. (2) A purgative agent that causes evacuation of the bowels.

cat's claw: Derived from the bark of a thick, slow-growing vine that encircles trees in the Peruvian rain forest. This herb is believed to help correct nutritional imbalances created by digestive blockages because of its ability to cleanse the intestinal tract. It is also believed to boost the immune system.

cat-scratch disease: An infectious disease which is transmitted by the bite or scratch of a cat. It is caused by *Pasteurella multocida*.

The disease is characterized by the formation of an abscess at the site of infection followed by enlargement of nearby lymph nodes.

cavitary lesion: (1) A circumscribed area of tissue altered by disease and characterized by the formation of a cavity. (2) Any lesion characterized by cavitation (internal or central necrosis, e.g., cavitary tuberculous).

cavitation: (1) Formation of a cavity. (2) A cavity.

CBC: *See* COMPLETE BLOOD COUNT.

CBO: *See* COMMUNITY-BASED ORGANIZATION.

CCA: *See* CITIZENS COMMISSION ON AIDS.

CCBC: *See* COUNCIL OF COMMUNITY BLOOD CENTERS.

CDC: *See* CENTERS FOR DISEASE CONTROL AND PREVENTION.

CDC National AIDS Clearinghouse (NAC): *See* CDC NATIONAL PREVENTION INFORMATION NETWORK.

CDC National Prevention Information Network (NPIN): Created for the purpose of disseminating information concerning the acquired immunodeficiency syndrome, the Clearinghouse distributes free educational materials, maintains a database for service providers, provides information concerning clinical trials, answers basic reference questions, and houses a resources center for visitors. Formerly called the National AIDS Information Clearinghouse and National AIDS Clearinghouse. CDC National Preventive Information Network, P.O. Box 6003, Rockville, MD 20849. Telephone: (800) 458-5231; TTY (800) 243-7012; Fax: (888) 282-7681.

cefotaxime: (1) A broad-spectrum antibiotic. (2) A third generation cephalosporin that is a semisynthetic derivative of cephamycin and is effective against gram-negative organisms that have the ability to resist certain types of antibiotics such as penicillin.

CEH: *See* NATIONAL CENTER FOR ENVIRONMENTAL HEALTH.

celiac disease: Disease of the intestinal system found almost exclusively in individuals who are sensitive to gluten and gliadin, two proteins found in wheat. Symptoms include weight loss, bloating, and diarrhea. *See* CELIAC DISEASE and SPRUE.

celibacy: *See* ABSTINENCE.

cell-mediated immunity: The immune response that arises from the interaction of an antigen and specialized lymphocytes, such as T cells. These responses include delayed hypersensitivity, defense against some bacteria, fungi, and viruses, and graft rejection. *Also called* CELLULAR IMMUNITY.

cellular immunity: (1) Immunity mediated by *T lymphocytes*. (2) T-cell mediated immune functions that need cell interactions (e.g., the destruction of infected cells). *Also called* CELL-MEDIATED IMMUNITY.

Center for Environmental Health (CEH): *See* NATIONAL CENTER FOR ENVIRONMENTAL HEALTH.

Center for Infectious Diseases (CID): *See* NATIONAL CENTER FOR INFECTIOUS DISEASES.

Center for Information Technology (CIT): One of the Centers of the National Institutes of Health, CIT incorporates powerful computer technology into all the biomedical programs and administrative procedures of the NIH through conducting computational bioscientific research, developing computer systems for biomedical needs, and providing computer facilities to the NIH campus. National Institutes of Health, Building 12A, Room 1011, 12 South Drive, Bethesda MD 20892. Telephone: (301) 496-6203. E-mail is available directly from the Web site, <http://www.cit.nih.gov/>.

Center for Mental Health Services (CMHS/SAMHSA): CMHS leads federal efforts both to treat and prevent mental illness. Established in 1992, CMHS is one of three centers that perform the work of the Substance Abuse and Mental Health Services Administration, Department of Health and Human Services, P.O. Box 42490, Washington, DC 20015. Telephone: (800) 789-2647; TDD: (301) 443-9006; Fax: (301) 984-8796. Both e-mail and Spanish language materials are available directly from the Web site, <http://www.mentalhealth.org/cmhs/index.htm>.

Center for Scientific Review (CSR): One of the centers of the National Institutes of Health (NIH), CSR is the office responsible for overseeing and initiating peer review of all NIH grant and award processes. National Institutes of Health, 6701 Rockledge Drive, Bethesda MD 20892. Telephone: (301) 435-1099. Both e-mail and

Spanish language materials are available directly from the Web site, <http://www.csr.nih.gov/>.

Center for Substance Abuse Prevention (CSAP/SAMHSA): CSAP leads federal efforts to prevent alcohol and other drug abuse among all citizens of the United Sates. CSAP is one of three centers that perform the work of the Substance Abuse and Mental Health Services Administration. Center for Substance Abuse Prevention, 5600 Fishers Lane, Rockwall II, Rockville, MD 20857. Telephone: (301) 443-0365. E-mail is available directly from the Web site, <http://www.samhsa.gov/csap/index.htm>.

Center for Substance Abuse Treatment (CSAT/SAMHSA): CSAT leads federal efforts to improve alcohol and other drug abuse treatment programs and to increase their availability to individuals in need. Additionally, CSAT conducts HIV/AIDS outreach programs that target high-risk substance abusers and their sexual partners. CSAT is one of three centers that perform the work of the Substance Abuse and Mental Health Services Administration. Telephone: (800) 662-4357 (hotline for referrals for drug and alcohol treatment). E-mail is available directly from the Web site, <http://www.samhsa.gov/csat/csat.htm>.

Centers for Disease Control and Prevention (CDC): The federal agency operating under the U.S. Department of Health and Human Services, Public Health Service which is responsible for protecting the public health of the nation by instituting measures for the prevention and control of diseases, epidemics, and public health emergencies. Founded in 1946, it is located at Centers for Disease Control, Department of Health and Human Services, Public Health Service, 1600 Clifton Road N.E., Atlanta, GA 30333. Telephone: (404) 639-33311 or toll-free (800) 311-3435. E-mail is available directly from the Web site, <http://www.cdc.gov/>.

central nervous system (CNS): The part of the body consisting of the brain and spinal cord, along with their nerves and ends of nerve fibers, that controls voluntary and involuntary muscles. It includes control of consciousness and mental functioning, sensory organs, and skeletal muscles.

central spinal fluid (CSF): *See* CEREBROSPINAL FLUID.

cerebrospinal fluid: The watery liquid which serves as a buffer to protect the brain and spinal cord from physical impact. *Also called* CENTRAL SPINAL FLUID or CSF.

cerebrovascular accident (CVA): A general term applied to conditions concerning the blood vessels of the brain that accompany either ischemic (caused by a lack of blood supply) or hemorrhagic (caused by the escape of large quantities of blood) lesions. *Also called* APOPLEXY or STROKE.

cervical cancer: Cancer of the cervix uteri.

cervical secretion: Any material produced by the cervix uteri from the blood.

cervix: (1) The neck, or part of an organ resembling a neck such as a column. (2) The narrow, outer end of the uterus.

cervix dysplasia: Presence of precancerous lesions in cervical tissue.

cervix neoplasm: *See* CERVICAL CANCER.

cervix uteri: The neck of the uterus.

chamomile: An herb derived from plants of the composite family with strong-smelling foliage, especially a plant whose dried daisy-like flower heads have been used in a medicinal tea. Believed to be an effective cleanser and toner of the digestive tract. Also believed to aid in calming the nerves.

chancre: The primary ulcer of syphilis, usually hard and painless, which appears at the point at which the infection enters the body. The lesion begins as an erosion or papule which is red or raw in color. It exudes fluid and continues to indurate. The sore heals without scarring. Syphilis is highly contagious during the chancre stage.

chapparal: An herb derived from the common desert shrub *Laurea tridentata*. It is believed to be effective in healing skin blemishes, acne, arthritis, and allergies. It is also believed to act as a natural antibiotic within the body.

charbon: *See* ANTHRAX.

chelation therapy: Therapy of heavy metal poisoning, using agents which sequester the metal from organs or tissues and bind it firmly within the ring structure of a new compound which can be eliminated from the body.

chemistry: The science dealing with the composition and properties of substances, and with the reactions by which substances are produced from or converted into other substances.

chemotaxis: The movement of cells in response to a chemical signal or stimulus (e.g., the movement of macrophages to the site of an inflammatory reaction).

chemotherapy: The treatment of disease by chemical reagents that have a toxic effect upon the disease-causing microorganism.

chest radiograph: An x-ray film of the chest cavity, taken for the purpose of making a definitive observation or measurement.

child: Any human between infancy and puberty.

child abuse: Mistreatment of children in a family, institution, or other setting. May be physical, emotional, verbal, sexual, or a combination of these.

Child Nutrition: Operated through the Food and Nutrition Service of the Department of Agriculture, the Child Nutrition Program provides support for children to eat nutritious food at school, day care, after school, and summer programs. United States Department of Agriculture, 14th and Independence, S.W., Washington, DC 20250. Telephone: Using the Web site, look under the state for which information is desired. Full information, including telephone and fax numbers, is included. E-mail is available directly from the Web site, <http://fns.usda.gov/cnd/>.

Chinese cucumber: *See* GLQ-223.

Chinese traditional medicine: A system of traditional medicine which is based on the beliefs and practices of the Chinese culture. Examples include acupuncture, herbal medicine, and yin-yang. *See also* ORIENTAL TRADITIONAL MEDICINE and KAMPO MEDICINE.

chiropractic: The science and art of restoring or maintaining health, practiced by a licensed professional, based on the theory that disease is caused by interference with nerve function, and employing manipulation of the body joints, especially of the spine, in seeking to restore normal nerve function.

Chlamydia: (1) A genus of bacteria that cause a variety of diseases in humans and other animals. (2) A genus of obligate, intracellular parasites that cause a variety of diseases in humans and animals. One species *Chlamydia trachomatis* has been recognized as the causative agent of a major sexually transmitted and perinatal infection, with genital infections caused by *Chlamydia trachomatis* being the most common sexually transmitted disease in the United States.

chlamydia: Any member of the genus *Chlamydia.*

chloramphenicol: A synthetic, broad-spectrum antibiotic which was originally isolated from *Streptomyces venezuelae.* It appears as elongated, needle-shaped crystals, and is whitish, grayish, or yellowish in color. It is especially useful in the treatment of typhus and other rickettsial infections, shigellosis, typhoid fever (for which it is the primary antibiotic for treatment), and salmonellosis (an opportunistic infectious complication of AIDS). In the treatment of bacterial infections, chloramphenicol may be administered orally or applied topically. It is administered orally in the treatment of rickettsial infections. The trade names are Chloromycetin and Chloroptic. *See also* RICKETTSIA.

Chloromycetin: *See* CHLORAMPHENICOL.

Chloroptic: *See* CHLORAMPHENICOL.

cholera: An acute infection of the small intestine, characterized by vomiting and painless, watery diarrhea, which results in the depletion of fluids and electrolytes, dehydration, muscular cramps, faint high-pitched voice, and collapse. Cholera is spread by feces-contaminated food and water. It is common in India and Southeast Africa, spreading periodically to other parts of the world.

cholesterol: A white, crystalline sterol, found in animal fats and oils, in bile, blood brain tissue, milk, egg yolk, myelin sheaths of nerve fibers, the liver, kidneys, and adrenal glands. It constitutes a large part of the most frequently occurring type of gallstones and occurs in atheroma of the arteries, in various cysts, and in cancerous tissue. Most of the body's cholesterol is synthesized in the liver, but some is absorbed from the diet.

choline: Considered to be a vitamin of the B complex, it is the basic constituent of lecithin and prevents the deposition of fat in the liver; facilitates the movement of fats in the cells; helps regulate the kidneys, liver, and gallbladder; and is essential for the synaptic transmission of nerve impulses.

choline magnesium trisalicylate: An anitarthritic that is a combination of choline salicylate and magnesium salicylate.

chorioid: *See* CHOROID.

chorioidea: *See* CHOROID.

chorioretinitis: Inflammation of the choroid and retina. *Also called* RETINOCHOROIDITIS.

choroid: The thin, dark brown, vascular coat of the eye which extends from the ora serrata to the optic nerve. It consists of blood vessels and connective tissue which furnish the blood supply to the retina. *Also called* CHORIOID, CHORIOIDEA, and CHOROIDEA.

choroidea: *See* CHOROID.

chromium: A trace element that plays a role in glucose metabolism and is considered essential in nutrition.

chronic: (1) Persisting over a long period of time. (2) Designating a disease exhibiting a slow progression. (3) The opposite of acute.

chronic ambulatory peritoneal dialysis: A treatment for kidney failure. Dialysis prolonged over a period of time in which warm, sterile, chemical solutions are perfused through the lining of the peritoneal cavity in order to remove toxic substances from the body. The patient is not confined to bed, and the procedure is repeated usually several times daily for as long as kidney function remains severely impaired.

chronic fatigue syndrome: A distinctive syndrome characterized by chronic fatigue, mild fever, lymphademopathy, headache, myalgia, arthralgia, depression, and memory loss. It may be caused by Epstein-Barr and other herpesviruses.

chronic hyperplastic candidiasis: Infection of the skin or mucous membrane with a species of *Candida* that causes a slow, excessive proliferation of normal cells in the normal tissue arrangement of the infected organ.

chronic mucocutaneous candidiasis: A clinical syndrome characterized by development, usually in infancy or childhood, of a chronic, often widespread candidiasis of skin, nails, and mucous membranes. It may be secondary to one of the immunodeficiency syndromes, inherited as an autosomal recessive trait, or associated with defects in cell-mediated immunity, endocrine disorders, dental stomatitis, or malignancy.

chronic infection: The invasion by, and multiplication of, a pathogenic agent in the body which persists over a prolonged period of time producing injurious effects.

chronic vaginal yeast infection: Infection of the vagina by any of several unicellular fungi of the genus *saccharomyces* that persists over a prolonged period of time.

CID: *See* CENTER FOR INFECTIOUS DISEASES.

cidofovir: (1) An antiviral drug that works against herpesviruses, including cytomegalovirus. (2) A nucleotide analogue that is a potent, selective inhibitor of human cytomegalovirus replication. Used to treat cytomegalovirus retinitis. Formerly known as HPMPC. The trade name is Vistide.

circumcision: (1) The removal of all or part of the foreskin of a male. (2) Incision of the fold of the skin over the glans clitoridis of a female.

CIT: *See* CENTER FOR INFORMATION TECHNOLOGY.

Citizens Commission on AIDS (CCA): Founded in 1987, this organization consisted of executives, leaders, and officials from the public and private sector concerned with the impact of HIV and AIDS on society. It sought to study and develop policies regarding the epidemic and to address the various ethical, moral, and legal aspects associated with the disease. The project ended in 1991 with the production of a final report.

citrovorum factor: *See* FOLINIC ACID.

civil rights: The freedom and liberty guaranteed to all citizens of the United States under the 13th, 14th, 15th, and 19th Amendments to the Constitution of the United States and by subsequent acts of Congress (i.e., equal treatment for all people).

Civil Rights Division: The Civil Rights Division of the Department of Justice is charged with enforcing all federal civil rights statutes that prohibit exclusion and discrimination and with educating the public about civil rights in order to promote equality and fairness for all. Particularly relevant to HIV/AIDS concerns are the Criminal Section, the Disability Rights Section, the Employment Litigation Section, and the Housing and Civil Enforcement Section. Office of the Assistant Attorney General, P.O. Box 65808, Washington, DC 20035. Telephone: (202) 514-2151; TDD: (202) 514-0716; Fax: (202) 514-0293. E-mail is available directly from the Web site, <http://www.usdoj.gov/crt/>.

clarithromycin: A semi-synthetic macrolide antibiotic; derivative of erythranycin.

Cleocin: *See* CLINDAMYCIN.

clindamycin: An antibiotic which is effective against gram-positive bacteria and some anaerobic infections. It has been used effectively to treat chorioretinitis; it has also been suggested that clindamycin used in conjunction with other drugs such as pyrimethamine may be successful treatment for infection with Toxoplasma gondii in some patients. The trade name is Cleocin.

clinical trial: A carefully designed and administered investigation of the effects of a new drug on human subjects. The purpose of a trial is to establish the clinical efficacy, safety, and pharmacologic effects of the substance. This is the process through which new drugs must pass in order to be approved by the United States Food and Drug Administration. *See also* PARALLEL TRACK.

clinical trial protocol: An explicit, detailed plan for a medical experiment.

clofazimine: An antibacterial which is used in the treatment of leprosy and tuberculosis.

clomipramine: A tricyclic antidepressant that selectively inhibits the uptake of serotonin to the brain. It is readily absorbed from the gastrointestinal tract and demethylated in the liver from its primary active metabolite, desmethylclomipramime.

clonazepam: An anticonvulsant used for several types of seizures.

clone: (1) The genetically identical offspring of cells, organisms, or plants propagated through asexual reproduction from a single parent. (2) The process of forming a clone.

cloning: The process of forming a clone.

closed-mouth kissing: Touching or caressing with the lips, without parting one's lips or opening one's mouth.

clothing exchange: A social service program where clothing is given to those in need.

clotrimazole: A broad-spectrum, antifungal drug used in the treatment of candidiasis and tinea. It is applied topically to the affected area of the skin, or intravaginally in the treatment of vulvovaginal candidiasis. Trade names include Gyne-Lotrimin, Lotrimin, and Mycelex G.

CMHS/SAMHSA: *See* CENTER FOR MENTAL HEALTH SERVICES.

CMV retinitis: *See* CYTOMEGALOVIRUS RETINITIS.

Cnidosporidia: *See* MICROSPORIDA.

CNS: *See* CENTRAL NERVOUS SYSTEM.

cobalamin: The cobalt-containing complex common to all members of the vitamin B12 group.

cocaine: A crystalline alkaloid obtained from the leaves of the shrub *Erythroxylon coca* and other *Erythroxylon* species. Cocaine may be used as a narcotic anesthetic when applied topically to mucous membranes. When administered for nonmedical use, it is classed as a drug of abuse. It may also be produced synthetically. *Also called* BLOW, COKE, and TOOT.

Coccidia: A large order of parasitic protozoa found in both vertebrates and invertebrates. They generally infect epithelial cells of the intestine and associated glands, and are the causative agent of coccidiosis.

Coccidioides: (1) A genus of fungi found in the soils of the southwestern United States that frequently infect persons with AIDS from this area. (2) A genus of imperfect, pathogenic fungi with but a single species, *Coccidioides immitis*. *Coccidioides immitis* is the causative agent of coccidioidomycosis. *See also* COCCIDIOIDOMYCOSIS.

Coccidioides immitis: See COCCIDIOIDES.

coccidioidomycosis: A fungal disease caused by infection with *Coccidioides immitis.* It exists in two forms: primary (an acute, self-limiting disease involving the respiratory system) and secondary or progressive (a chronic, severe, virulent, tumor-containing disease that may involve most any part of the body). *Also called* VALLEY FEVER.

coccidiosis: A disease-producing condition caused by infection with *coccidia* generally affecting the intestines. In humans, symptoms include watery, mucous stools; anorexia; and nausea. *See also* ISOPORA BELLI INFECTION.

code-blue status: Directions to employ active and aggressive cardiopulmonary resuscitation in the event of the apparent cessation of life.

codeine: An opioid analgesic related to morphine but with less potent analgesic properties and mild sedative effects. It also acts centrally to suppress cough.

cofactor: An element or principle which acts in conjunction with another. Generally, the cofactor must be present for the other to function.

cognition: The mental process by which one becomes aware of thought and perception, including reasoning, judgment, and memory.

coke: *See* COCAINE.

colitis: Inflammation of the colon.

colon: The part of the large intestine extending from the cecum to the rectum.

colonic irrigation: Washing out of the colon.

coloproctitis: *See* PROCTOCOLITIS.

color therapy: A form of phototherapy using color to influence health and to treat various physical or mental disorders. The color rays may be in the visible or invisible spectrum and can be administered through colored lights or applied mentally through suggestion.

colposcopy: Use of a specially designed, lighted microscope (colposcope) to examine vaginal, cervical, or anal tissues, especially for biopsy following an abnormal Pap smear. In HIV-positive women, colposcopy is preferred to Pap smear as a diagnostic tool for cervical cancer.

combination therapy: Use of two or more drugs to treat a condition or ailment. May be used to take advantage of potent drug interactions or to forestall drug resistance that is often the result of monotherapy.

combined modality therapy: *See* COMBINATION THERAPY.

combivir: An antiretroviral tablet consisting of lamivudine and zidovudine.

comfrey: Any of a group of a genus of European plants of the borage family, with rough, hairy leaves and small blue, purplish, or yellow flowers. It is believed that comfrey aids in healing respiratory ailments, anemia, arthritis, fractures, mucous membranes, lungs, and wounds. It is also thought to soothe the gastrointestinal tract, aid in cell proliferation, help the pancreas in regulating blood sugar levels, help promote the secretion of pepsin, and generally aid in digestion.

coming out: Disclosure by an individual of a personal issue (e.g., homosexual orientation or injection drug use) either to close associates or, in the case of a famous person, to the world at large.

Community Acquired Immune Deficiency Syndrome (CAIDS): One of a group of names initially used to denote the acquired immunodeficiency syndrome. *See also* GAY-RELATED IMMUNE DEFICIENCY, ACQUIRED COMMUNITY IMMUNE DEFICIENCY SYNDROME, and ACQUIRED IMMUNODEFICIENCY SYNDROME.

Community Research Initiative (CRI): The first community organization to do actual drug research on possible treatments for AIDS and the various diseases and opportunistic infections that accompany it. The program is now part of the People With AIDS Coalition. Community Research Initiative, People With AIDS Coalition, 31 W. 26th Street, New York, NY 10011. Telephone: (212) 532-0290.

Community-based organization (CBO): Any organization that is created and administered at the community level. CBOs typically are not affiliated with academic institutions or government agencies.

Compassionate Use: A program developed by the Food and Drug Administration to supply experimental drugs to the seriously ill who have no other alternatives. Compassionate Use allows a drug to be dispensed in lieu of following the standard protocol for FDA approval (clinical trials).

Compazine: *See* PROCHLORPERAZINE.

competence: The condition or quality to manage one's affairs; the ability to fulfill one's needs.

complement fixation test: A procedure used to detect antigens or antibodies. Complement fixation involves the action of a complement upon reaction with immune complexes containing complement-fixing antibodies. The complement is rendered inactive during the uniting of antibody, antigen, and complement (fixation of complement). This is the basis for determining the presence of antigens or antibodies.

complete blood count (CBC): A measurement of the hemoglobin, hematocrit, and erythrocyte indices by counting the number of leukocytes and erythrocytes per unit volume in a sample of venous blood.

complication: A second disease or abnormal condition occurring during the course of a primary disease.

Compound Q: *See* GLQ-223.

computed tomographic scan: *See* COMPUTERIZED AXIAL TOMOGRAPHIC SCAN.

computer bulletin boards: *See* ELECTRONIC BULLETIN BOARDS.

computerized axial tomographic scan (CAT scan): (1) A noninvasive procedure for diagnosing disorders of the body, especially in the soft tissues. (2) A noninvasive procedure employing special techniques of roentgenography in which transverse planes of tissue are swept by an x-ray beam and the variance in absorption is recorded on a magnetic disk, processed on a minicomputer, and used to produce a precise reconstruction of that area. This technique is more sensitive than traditional radiographic procedures, and has been very successful in diagnostic studies of the brain. *Also called* CAT SCAN and COMPUTED TOMOGRAPHIC SCAN.

condition: A state of health.

condom: A thin, flexible sheath or cover for the penis, worn during sexual intercourse to prevent semen from entering the mouth, anus, or vagina and to prevent venereal disease. Only those condoms made of latex prevent transmission of the human immunodeficiency virus. *See also* FEMALE CONDOM.

condom distribution program: Any social service program distributing condoms to foster safer sex and deter the spread of HIV infection.

condom efficacy: The ability of a condom to produce its desired effect, to prevent the comingling of body fluids during sexual intercourse.

condyloma acuminatum: (1) A wart occurring on the area around the anus or external genitals. (2) A papilloma caused by a virus, and occurring on the mucous membrane or skin of the external genitals or perianal region. It is infectious and autoinoculable. Although the lesions are usually small in number, they may cluster to form a cauliflower-like mass. *Also called* VENEREAL WART. *See also* HUMAN PAPILLOMAVIRUS and ANAL WART.

confidentiality: The privacy afforded information entrusted to health care and other professionals (lawyers, clergy, etc.) concerning a patient (e.g., test results). This privileged information cannot be divulged to a third party without the patient's consent, unless it is deemed injurious to public health under certain circumstances.

congenital: Existing at birth; present at birth.

congestive cardiomyopathy: A syndrome characterized by cardiac enlargement and congestive heart failure. It probably represents the end result of many forms of myocardial damage produced by a variety of toxic, metabolic, or infectious agents.

congestive heart failure: *See* CONGESTIVE CARDIOMYOPATHY.

conservatorship: The responsibility or rank of custodian, guardian, or protector.

contact tracing: To follow the track of individuals who have been recently exposed to a contagious disease; implies informing those individuals who may have been exposed. *See also* PARTNER NOTIFICA-TION.

contraceptive: An agent, device, method, or process which works to prevent conception. Common classes include chemicals (spermicides, birth control pills), natural (abstinence or rhythm), physical or barrier (condoms, IUDs, sponges, caps, or diaphragms), and permanent (tubal ligation and vasectomy).

control group: A standard against which observations or conclusions may be compared for the purpose of verifying the results of an experiment.

controlled clinical trial: Clinical trials involving one or more test treatments, at least one control treatment, specified outcome measures for evaluating the studied intervention, and a basis-free method for assigning patients to the test treatment. The treatment may be drugs, devices, or procedures studied for diagnostic, therapeutic, or prophylactic effectiveness. Control measures include placebos, active medicines, no-treatment, dosage forms and regimens, historical comparisons, etc.

Coomb's test: A procedure used to detect antiglobulins in the red cell. It is used in diagnosing various hemolytic anemias.

Coomb's-positive anemia: Any type of anemia detected by a Coomb's test.

coping therapies: Any of a group of therapeutic mechanisms designed to assist individuals in dealing with problems or troubles.

copper: A mineral necessary for the absorption and utilization of iron. Helps oxidize vitamin C and works with it to form elastin, a chief component of the elastin muscle fibers throughout the body. Also aids in the formation of red blood cells and helps proper bone formation and maintenance.

coronary disease: A form of insufficient blood supply to the heart muscle caused by a decreased capacity of the coronary vessels.

correctional institution: Any facility charged with carrying out punishment for the purpose of altering behavior (e.g., juvenile detention center or prison).

corticosteroid: Any of the hormonal steroids obtained from the adrenal cortex. Divided as to their biological activity into 3 main groups: glucocorticoids (those affecting carbohydrate, fat, and protein metabolism); mineralocorticoids (those influencing the regulation of electrolyte and water balance); and androgen (those affecting the development of male characteristics). Corticosteroids do not initiate activity, but allow for many biochemical reactions to proceed at optimal rates.

cortisone: A hormone found in the cortex of the adrenal gland and also produced synthetically. It possesses properties that make it useful in the treatment of various allergic, inflammatory, and neoplastic diseases.

Cotinazin: *See* ISONIAZID.

cotton-wool spots: Fluffy white lesions with obvious boundaries that appear on the eye. These are generally not associated with hemorrhages and should be differentiated from cytomegalovirus retinitis since they are generally asymptomatic, may subside voluntarily, and generally have a favorable prognosis.

Council of Community Blood Centers (CCBC): Founded in 1962, this organization comprises nonprofit, independent blood centers licensed by the federal government and serving specific geographic areas. It serves to ensure the maintenance and provision of an optimal supply of blood and blood products. The CCBC conducts research, compiles statistics, and serves as a liaison to various organizations interested in the storage of blood. In 1998, the name was changed to America's Blood Centers. America's Blood Centers, 725 15th Street N.W., Suite 700, Washington, DC 20005. Telephone: (202) 393-5725.

counseling: The provision of advice or guidance to a patient by health care and other professionals. Counseling is often recommended to assist a patient in coping with stress or working through various types of problems.

countertransference: A psychiatrist's, psychologist's, or psychotherapist's conscious or unconscious emotional reaction to a patient.

cranial nerve disease: *See* CRANIAL NERVE PALSY.

cranial nerve palsy: The temporary or permanent loss of sensation, or ability to control movement, in the twelve pairs of nerves that originate in the brain.

craniofacial feature: The appearance, form, or shape of the face and the skeleton of the head.

creatinine: The anhydride of creatine. It is found in blood, muscle, and especially urine, where measurement of its excretion is used to evaluate kidney function.

cremation: The procedure of burning a dead body to ashes.

Creutzfeldt-Jakob disease: A rare, transmissible, usually fatal disease that causes degeneration of the brain. It is accompanied by progressive dementia and sometimes wasting of the muscles, tremor, and spastic speech impairment. The way the disease is acquired naturally is unknown; however, human to human transmission has occurred by parenteral administration of growth hormone prepared from cadaveric human pituitary glands, cadaveric dura mater graft, implantation of contaminated electroencephalographic electrodes, and corneal transplantation. A variant form of Creutzfeldt-Jakob disease appears to be closely related to the clinical and pathological manifestations of Kuru disease. This variant form has been related to bovine spongiform encephalopathy (more commonly known as Mad Cow Disease).

CRI: *See* COMMUNITY RESEARCH INITIATIVE.

Criminal Section of the Civil Rights Division: This arm of the Department of Justice is a trial section staffed by attorneys who prosecute cases of national significance involving the deprivation of personal liberties that transcend the jurisdictions of state or local authorities. Cases may include acts of violence based on ethnicity, hate crimes, violation of involuntary servitude laws that protect migrant workers, and other cases where perpetrators have sought to abridge personal freedoms guaranteed by the U. S. Constitution. Criminal Section of the Civil Rights Division, P.O. Box 66018, Washington, DC 20035. Telephone: (202) 514-3204; Web site, <http://www.usjoj.gov/>.

crisis intervention: The process of alleviating or terminating an unstable emotional or mental period in a person's life through problem resolution. Many telephone hot lines (e.g., suicide prevention hotlines or AIDS hotlines) function as crisis intervention services. These are generally staffed by professionals or paraprofessionals trained in the medical or social sciences.

Crixivan: *See* INDINAVIR.

cryptococcal meningitis: A type of meningitis caused by *Cryptococcus neoformans*. It is a common opportunistic infection among AIDS patients and can be fatal if not treated. *See also* CRYPTOCCOSIS.

cryptococcosis: (1) A serious opportunistic fungal infection by *Cryptococcus neoformans* that may involve several places in the body. (2) A systemic infection by *Cryptococcus neoformans* which may involve the skin, lungs, or any organ of the body, but has a predilection for the brain and meninges. The cutaneous form is characterized by abscesses or lesions. In the generalized form, the central nervous system is the primary target for attack. This is marked by dizziness, headache, stiffness of the neck muscles, and vertigo. If untreated, coma and respiratory failure result. *Also called* BUSSE-BUSCHKE DISEASE and TORULOPSOSIS.

Cryptococcus: A genus of asexual, pathogenic, yeast-like fungi. It is the causative agent of cryptococcosis.

cryptosporidiosis: An enteric (gastrointestinal) disease caused by infection with protozoa of the genus *cryptosporidium* and characterized by diarrhea. This disease is not uncommon in hoofed animals. Human occurrence appears in both the immunocompetent and immunocompromised. Among the immunocompetent, infection is largely among those working with infected animals. For these individuals, diarrhea is accompanied by abdominal cramps and lasts up to a month. The malady is self-limiting and there is no therapy. The disease is much more serious in the immunocompromised patient, and often results in death. Diarrhea is prolonged and debilitating; it is accompanied by abdominal cramps, fever, and weight loss.

Cryptosporidium: A genus of parasitic, coccidian protozoa. They inhabit the intestinal tracts of various birds, mammals, and reptiles. In humans, infection may cause diarrhea. This is especially true for the immunocompromised patient. *See also* CRYPTOSPORIDIOSIS.

CSAP/SAMHSA: *See* CENTER FOR SUBSTANCE ABUSE PREVENTION.

CSAT/SAMHSA: *See* CENTER FOR SUBSTANCE ABUSE TREATMENT.

CSF: *See* CEREBROSPINAL FLUID.

CSR: *See* CENTER FOR SCIENTIFIC REVIEW.

culture: (1) The propagation of microorganisms or of living tissue cells in special media that are conducive to their growth. (2) The ideas, beliefs, and customs of a group of people that are transferred or communicated to subsequent generations.

Cumulated Index Medicus: An annual index, updated monthly, to biomedical literature. It is produced by the National Library of Medicine, and citations are gleaned from the vast collection of journals collected by NLM. *Also called* INDEX MEDICUS. MEDLINE is the electronic counterpart. National Library of Medicine, 8600 Rockville Pike, Bethesda, MD 20894. Telephone: (301) 594-5983 or toll-free (888) 346-3656.

cunnilingus: Sexual activity in which the female genitalia are stimulated with the tongue and mouth.

curcumin: An orange-yellow, crystalline substance that is the coloring principle of turmeric. Curcumin appears to possess a spectrum of pharmacological properties, due primarily to its inhibitory effects on metabolic enzymes.

Cure AIDS Now (CAN): Founded in 1985, this organization seeks to educate the public as to the reality and gravity of the pandemic. It also functions as a support network for persons with AIDS and those interested in assisting with the fight to stop the spread of HIV. CAN coordinates resources donated by private and corporate sources to create and execute AIDS assistance programs. Cure AIDS Now, 2240 S. Dixie Highway, Coconut Grove, FL 33133. Telephone: (305) 856-TEST.

cutaneous abnormalities: A malformation or deformity of the skin.

cutaneous candidiasis: Candidiasis of the skin. *See also* KAPOSI'S SARCOMA.

cutaneous Kaposi's sarcoma: Kaposi's sarcoma of the skin.

CVA: *See* CEREBROVASCULAR ACCIDENT.

cycloserine: A broad-spectrum antibiotic, administered orally, and shown to be effective in the treatment of tuberculosis. It is also effective against various gram-positive and gram-negative bacteria, including some that infect the pulmonary system and urinary tract. The trade name is Seromycin.

cyclosporine A: An immunosuppressive and antifungal drug used to prevent rejection in organ transplant recipients. The trade name is Sandimmune.

Cylert: *See* PEMOLINE.

cystine: A nonessential amino acid. It functions as an antioxidant and is believed to be a powerful aid to the body in protecting against radiation and pollution. It is believed to help slow the aging process, deactivate free radicals, and neutralize toxins. It is necessary for skin formation and is present in both hair and skin.

cytodiagnosis: Diagnosis of disease based on the examination of cells.

cytokine: (1) A substance that is released by a cell population when it is stimulated by a specific antigen. (2) A nonantibody protein that is released when a specific antigen interacts with a cell population. Cytokines serve as the substance situated between cells which enable the generation and propagation amplification of a response (e.g., T lymphocytes emit cytokines, allowing for an immune response).

cytomegalic inclusion disease: Any of a group of diseases caused by infection with the cytomegalovirus, and marked by the presence of bodies in the cytoplasm of infected cells. Infection can occur congenitally, postnatally, via respiratory droplets, tissue, or blood donation, or through sexual intercourse. Included in this group is an infectious mononucleosis-like syndrome that occurs in recipients of multiple blood transfusions and previously well individuals, and a disseminated infection in immunosuppressed or immunocompromised patients that is fatal.

cytomegalovirus (CMV): One of a group of highly species-specific herpesviruses that infect humans, monkeys, or rodents. In humans, cytomegalovirus is found in the salivary glands. It may cause a variety of clinical syndromes that are collectively known as cytomegalic inclusion disease. *Also called* SALIVARY GLAND VIRUS.

cytomegalovirus retinitis (CMV retinitis): Inflammation of the retina, which may result in blindness, due to infection with the cytomegalovirus.

cytosine: A base that is part of both DNA and RNA.

cytotoxicity: The degree to which an agent possesses a specific action which is destructive to certain cells.

Cytovene: *See* GANCICLOVIR.

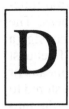

dance therapy: Use of dance or dance-like movements to promote healing and reduce stress.

dandelion: A common, yellow-flowered composite herb believed to be effective against gastrointestinal disturbance and dermatitis. Also acts as a diuretic.

dapsone: (1) A broad-spectrum antibacterial. (2) An antibacterial sulfone, administered orally and used in the treatment of leprosy, which inhibits or retards bacterial growth in a variety of gram-negative and gram-positive organisms. Also used in the treatment of dermatitis herpetiformis, and in the prophylaxis of falciparum malaria and *Pneumocystis carinii* pneumonia. *Also called* DIAMINODI-PHENYLSULFONE or DDS. The trade name is Avlosulfon.

dapsone/trimethoprim: Combination drug therapy using dapsone and trimethoprim. A common outpatient regimen for the treatment of *Pneumocystis carinii* pneumonia.

Daraprim: *See* PYRIMETHAMINE.

dating services: Organizations that take information from individuals and attempt to match them with other people in their files. Some services work only with HIV-positive persons.

ddC: *See* ZALCITABINE.

ddI: *See* DIDANOSINE.

DDS: *See* DAPSONE.

death: (1) The cessation of life. (2) The permanent cessation of all bodily functions. (3) The phase following dying. For legal purposes, death has been defined to include the irreversible cessation of cerebral function, spontaneous respiratory system function, and spontaneous circulatory system function.

death counseling: The providing of advice and guidance to a patient by a health professional concerning end of life issues. May also apply to individuals preparing for or coping with the loss of a loved one.

death with dignity: The concept of allowing a patient to die, rather than artificially prolonging life, that arose out of the ability of modern medical and technological advances to maintain vital functions in persons who may or may not regain consciousness. The patient (or the patient's family if he/she is unconscious) may sign a statement to prevent the artificial prolongation of life: "I request that I be allowed to die and not be kept alive by artificial means or heroic measures. I ask only that drugs be mercifully administered to me to alleviate terminal suffering even if they may hasten the moment of death."

Decadron: *See* DEXAMETHASONE.

decubitus ulcer: (1) A bed sore. (2) An ulceration of the skin due to prolonged pressure over the affected area in a patient allowed to lie still in the same position in bed too long. The tissue dies due to a lack of blood supply. Areas with prominent bones are at greatest risk. If not treated properly, the ulcer can progress to the deeper layers of the skin and may eventually affect the underlying muscle and bone.

definitive diagnosis: (1) A diagnosis established with certainty and without question. (2) The opposite of presumptive diagnosis.

dehydroepiandrosterone (DHEA): An androgenic substance present in urine. The level of this hormone in plasma decreases with age as well as with progression of HIV disease.

delavirdine: A potent non-nucleoside reverse transcriptase inhibitor with activity specific for HIV 1.

delirium: A state of mental confusion and disorder characterized by the inability to focus attention, disorientation, incoherent speech, sensory misperceptions, disturbance in motor skills, and memory impairment. Forms of delirium vary depending on the cause (infection, fever, drug overdose or side effect, shock, trauma, or metabolic disturbances).

delivered meals: Nutrition delivered to the homes of people unable to prepare meals for themselves. The federally subsidized Meals on Wheels as well as local programs such as God's Love We Deliver are examples of delivered meals.

deltacortisone: *See* PREDNISONE.

Deltasone: *See* PREDNISONE.

Demerol: *See* MEPERIDINE.

demography: The statistical and quantitative science dealing with the age, density, distribution, growth, size, and vital statistics of human populations.

demonstration: Activity, usually planned, designed to call the media and public attention to an issue. Demonstrations may include speakers, placards, and symbolic gestures (e.g., sending balloons aloft). Occasionally, heated exchanges lead to violence. One of the most famous demonstrations in the history of the AIDS epidemic occurred at the National Institutes of Health, Food and Drug Administration, when participants assumed control of the building and demanded drug treatments for HIV disease and opportunistic infections.

demyelinate: To remove or destroy the myelin sheath surrounding a nerve or nerves, interrupting the transmission of nerve impulses.

dendrite: One of the threadlike extensions of the cytoplasm of a neuron that comprise most of the receptive surface of a neuron, and conducts impulses to another nerve cell body.

denial: (1) A defense mechanism in which the existence of anxiety-producing realities are kept out of conscious awareness. (2) The refusal to admit the existence of something.

dental dam: Square of latex used during cunnilingus to protect partner from possible infection with a sexually transmitted disease.

dentistry: Preventive care, repair, and replacement of teeth.

deoxynojirimycin: A plant alkaloid that, in the laboratory, inhibits cell-to-cell spread and formation of nucleated protoplasmic mass induced by the human immunodeficiency virus.

deoxyribonucleic acid (DNA): A nucleic acid that makes up the genetic material of cellular organisms and DNA viruses. It is a complex protein, high in molecular weight, consisting of deoxyribose, phosphoric acid, and four bases [two purine (adenine and guanine) and two pyrimides (thymine and cytosine)]. It is bound by hydrogen bonds between the bases into double helical chains, forming the basic material in the chromosomes of the cell nucleus.

Department of Agriculture: Charged with enhancing the quality of life for all Americans by supporting the production of agriculture and working to reduce hunger in the United States and the world, the USDA operates several offices and programs relevant to HIV/ AIDS through their Nutrition Assistance Programs. Department of Agriculture, 14th and Independence, S.W., Washington, DC 20250. Telephone: (202) 720-2791; TDD: (202) 720-2600. E-mail is available directly from the Web site, <http://www.usda.gov/>.

Department of Defense: The DoD is charged with providing the military forces needed to deter war and to protect the security of the United States. The Department maintains military and health records for all active duty military personnel, and can assist with locating such personnel. OASD (PA) (Office of the Assistant Secretary of Defense/Public Affairs), 1400 Defense Pentagon, Room 1E757, Washington, DC 20301-1400. Telephone: (703) 697-5737. E-mail is available directly from the Web site, <http://www.defenselink.mil/>, which also includes postal mail addresses for the Secretary of Defense and other senior officials in the department.

Department of Education (ED): Established in 1979, the Department of Education administers more than 150 federal education programs including student loans, vocational training, and special education for the handicapped and disabled. The Department's Web site includes information about qualifications for disabilities education and help for children who lack health insurance. Department of Education, 400 Maryland Avenue, S.W., Washington, DC 20202. Telephone: (800) 872-5327 (page of toll-free numbers for ED programs is on Web site); TTY: (800) 437-0833; Fax: (202) 401-0689. E-mail is available directly from the Web site, <http://www.ed.gov/>.

Department of Health and Human Services (DHHS): The cabinet-level department of the federal executive branch most concerned with people and most involved with the Nation's human concerns. Department of Health and Human Services, 200 Independence Avenue, S.W., Washington, DC 20201. Telephone: (202) 619-0257 or toll-free (877) 696-6775. E-mail is available directly from the Web site, <http://www.hud.gov/>.

Department of Housing and Urban Development (HUD): HUD was established in 1965 as a successor to the Housing and Home Finance Agency, which had been created in 1947. The agency is responsible for promoting community development, administering fair housing laws, and providing affordable subsidies for housing.Deaprtment of Housing and Urban Development, 451 7th Street, S.W., Washington, DC 20410. Telephone: (800) 245-2691. E-mail is available directly from the Web site, <http://www.hud.gov/>.

Department of Justice (DOJ): Responsible for the supervision of federal district attorneys and marshals and federal penal institutions, DOJ attorneys also represent the United States in legal matters and provide legal advice to federal officials in the Executive Branch. The Federal Bureau of Investigation, Immigration and Naturalization Service, and the Civil Rights Division all operate through this department. Department of Justice, 950 Pennsylvania Avenue, N.W., Washington, DC 20530. Telephone: (202) 514-2000. E-mail is available directly from the Web site, <http://www.usdoj.gov/>.

Department of Labor (DOL): The Department of Labor administers and enforces legislative mandates and regulations that cover workers' wages, health and safety, and employment and pension rights. The DOL promotes equal employment opportunity; administers job training, unemployment insurance, and workers' compensation programs; strengthens collective bargaining initiatives; and collects, analyzes, and publishes labor and economic statistics. The Web site contains helpful information about the Health Insurance Portability Accountability Act of 1996. Branches of the DOL particularly relevant to HIV/AIDS include the Employment and Training Administration, the Occupational Safety and Health Administration, the Pension and Welfare Benefits Administration, the Veterans' Employment and Training Service, and the Women's Bureau. Department of Labor, Office of Public Affairs, 200 Constitution Avenue, N.W., Room S-1032, Washington, DC 20210. Telephone: (202) 693-4650. E-mail is available directly from the Web site, <http://www.dol.gov/>.

Department of Veterans' Affairs (VA): The VA administers insurance, health, education, vocational rehabilitation and counseling services, and burial information for all men and women who have served in the nation's armed forces. Department of Veteran's Affairs, 810 Vermont Avenue, N.W., Washington, DC 20420. Telephone: (800) 827-1000; TDD: (800) 829-4833. E-mail to state VA offices is available directly from the Web site, <http://www.va.gov/>.

deportation: Expulsion of aliens from a country. May or may not include transport to the country of origin.

depression: (1) A hollow or concave region. (2) A decrease or lowering of a functional activity or vital function. (3) A mental state denoted by an altered mood and characterized by feelings of despair, discouragement, guilt, hopelessness, helplessness, the inability to cope, low self-esteem, and sadness. Depression often results in withdrawal from those activities usually found to be pleasurable. It may also cause changes in eating patterns, energy, and sleep disturbances; it ranges from a general feeling of the blues through major clinical depression.

dermatitis: Inflammation of the skin.

dermatitis medicamentosa: *See* DRUG ERUPTION.

dermatologic disorder: Abnormal condition of the skin.

dermatology: Branch of biomedicine that specializes in the study of the skin.

Design Industries Foundation Fighting AIDS (DIFFA): Founded in 1984, this organization raises funds for people with AIDS. It supports patient care and services including education, housing, food, emergency assistance, legal advocacy, treatment, and research. The Foundation produces and distributes educational materials, and makes presentations and referrals. Design Industries Foundation Fighting AIDS, 150 W. 26th Street, Suite 602, New York, NY 10001. Telephone: (212) 727-3100.

Designated AIDS Center Program: A program created and implemented by the New York State Department of Health (funded by Medicaid to cover New York) to assist with the high cost of AIDS. It seeks to help by addressing the ways in which health care services are organized. *See also* AIDS HEALTH SERVICE PROGRAM, AIDS SERVICE DEMONSTRATION PROGRAM, and AIDS-SPECIFIC MEDICAID HOME AND COMMUNITY-BASED WAIVERS.

desipramine: An antidepressant. Trade names are Norpramin and Pertofrane.

desmopressin: A vasopressin analogue, with antidiuretic (water retention) properties, used in the treatment of diabetes insipidus. Also used to increase Factor VIII (the factor contributing to the intrinsic value of blood coagulation) for hemophiliacs or patients with von Willebrand's disease before surgery.

Desyrel: *See* TRAZODONE.

dexamethasone: A synthetic glucocorticoid drug used in treatment of conditions that respond generally to cortisone. Trade names are Decadron and SK-Dexamethasone.

Dexedrine: *See* DEXTROAMPHETAMINE.

dextran sulfate: (1) A potential treatment for HIV infection that proved to be ineffective. (2) A sulfated polysaccharide that showed promise as an antiviral treatment for HIV infection in vitro, but in a Phase I/II trial (*See* CLINICAL TRIAL) in San Francisco demonstrated no antiviral or clinical immunological efficacy.

dextroamphetamine: The d-form of amphetamine. It is a central nervous system stimulant and a sympathomimetic. It has also been used in the treatment of narcolepsy and attention deficit disorder and hyperactivity in children. Dextroamphetamine is also a psychotomimatic and a drug of abuse.

d4T: *See* STAVUDINE.

DHEA: *See* DEHYDROEPIANDROSTERONE.

DHPG: *See* GANCICLOVIR.

diabetes: *See* DIABETES MELLITUS.

diabetes insipidus: A metabolic disorder caused by damage to the neurohypophyseal system (the main portion of the posterior lobe of the pituitary gland). This results in deficient amounts of antidiuretic hormone (vasopressin) produced or released. As a result, the individual experiences uncontrollable excessive thirst and urination. It may be acquired, inherited, or of unknown origin.

diabetes mellitus: Usually referred to simply as diabetes, a chronic metabolic disorder caused by failure of the body to produce enough insulin or to use it appropriately. Two broad types of diabetes mellitus exist: Type 1, or juvenile-onset diabetes, in which the individual produces no insulin; much more common is non-insulin-dependent diabetes, which generally occurs in persons past the age of 40. *See also* INSULIN.

diacetylmorphine: A narcotic morphine derivative which appears as a white, crystalline powder. Because of its highly addictive nature, importation, use, or sale is illegal in the United States. *Also called* HEROIN.

diagnosis: The use of scientific methods to determine the cause and nature of a person's disease or illness.

diagnostic imaging: Use of one of the following technologies— X ray, ultrasound, magnetic resonance, or infrared—to examine a portion of the body as part of the procedure for determining the cause, nature, location, and extent of an individual's illness. *See also* X RAY, MAGNETIC RESONANCE IMAGING, and ULTRASOUND.

dialysis: The process of separating out materials in solution due to the difference in their rates of diffusion through a semipermeable membrane. *See also* HEMODIALYSIS AND PERITONEAL DIALYSIS.

diaminodiphenylsulfone: *See* DAPSONE.

diarrhea: A disturbance in bowel movements characterized by abnormal frequency and liquidity. Diarrhea is often related to a disturbance in the gastrointestinal system.

diarrhea-wasting syndrome: A term sometimes used to refer to diarrhea as commonly associated with HIV infection. The syndrome (diarrhea persisting for at least one month accompanied by unexplained weight loss of 10 percent of the premorbid weight) in conjunction with infection with the human immunodeficiency virus comprises an AIDS-defining illness.

diazepam: An anti-anxiety and sedative drug. Trade name is Valium.

didanosine (ddI): A nucleoside analogue similar to zidovudine. It has been approved by the Food and Drug Administration for treatment of adult and pediatric patients with advanced HIV infection, and who are intolerant to or significantly deteriorate while on AZT. Trade name is Videx.

dideoxycytidine (ddC): *See* ZALCITABINE.

dideoxyinosine: *See* DIDANOSINE.

diet: (1) Food substances of any consistency regularly consumed in the course of daily living. (2) Restriction of food substances in order to treat a disease (e.g., diabetes) or a temporary condition (e.g., following surgery). (3) Restriction or supplementation of food intake for the purpose of controlling weight.

diet therapy: Attempt to effect an improvement in a condition or in overall health and well-being through control of what one eats and drinks.

dietetics: Application of nutritional principles and data to the study of the kinds and quantities of food needed for health.

DIFFA: *See* DESIGN INDUSTRIES FOUNDATION FIGHTING AIDS.

differential diagnosis: The diagnostic approach which compares the symptoms of two or more similar diseases in order to determine which one the patient is suffering from.

Diflucan: *See* FLUCONAZOLE.

digital intercourse: Penetration and stimulation of the anus or vagina with a partner's fingers.

dihydroxypropoxymethyl (DHPG): *See* GANCICLOVIR.

diiodohydroxyquin: *See* IODOQUINOL.

Dilaudid: *See* HYDROMORPHONE.

dildo: An artificial, penis-shaped device used to promote sexual pleasure.

Dinacrin: *See* ISONIAZID.

Diodoquin: *See* IODOQUINOL.

dipstick test: A method to determine the presence of protein, glucose, or other substances in the urine using a chemically impregnated strip of paper.

Disability Rights Section of the Civil Rights Division: This arm of the Department of Justice protects the rights of persons with disabilities guaranteed under the Americans with Disabilities Act (ADA). Disability Rights Section of the Civil Rights Division, P.O. Box 66738, Washington, DC 20035. Telephone and TDD: (202) 307-0663; Fax: (202) 307-1198; Web site, <http://www.usdoj.gov/>.

disclosure issues: Circumstances surrounding the revelation of a socially unacceptable act, especially homosexuality, illicit drug use, abuse, and similar controversial topics. Adds an additional measure of stress to HIV-infected men or women who must reveal to families, friends, or themselves facts about their private lives.

discrimination: The process of differentiating, distinguishing, or excluding based on some characteristic or trait (e.g., race, religion, sexual orientation).

disinfection: The act of freeing from pathogenic organisms, or to render them inactive, by physical or chemical means. Generally used in reference to inanimate objects.

disseminated tuberculosis: The spread of Mycobacterium tuberculosis from the primary focus of infection through the blood or lymphatic system.

distal: Remote; away from the point of origin.

distal symmetric polyneuropathy (DSPN): A disease of the nerves that manifests as subacute onset of numbness or tingling in the fingers or toes. Early clinical signs are bilaterally depressed ankle reflex and impaired sensation in the toes. Approximately 35 percent of hospitalized AIDS patients are affected by DSPN.

diversity threshold: The point at which the immune system can no longer recognize and subdue all viral variants, given the enormous capacity for HIV to mutate. This theory is not universally accepted.

divorce: Legal dissolution of a marriage. Also, any other separation that is both permanent and immutable.

DMP 266: *See* EFAVIRENZ.

DNA: *See* DEOXYRIBONUCLEIC ACID.

DNA polymerase alpha: An enzyme essential to the life of a cell for its synthetic and repair functions.

DNA polymerase beta: An enzyme with repair functions in the life of a cell.

DNA polymerase gamma: An enzyme consisting of cells that contain small granules or rod-shaped structures found in differential staining of the cytoplasm.

DNCB: Chemical that stimulated a powerful immune response when applied to the skin. First suggested as a treatment for AIDS in the mid-1980s by a dermatologist, L. Bruce Mills, MD. Activists theorized that DNCB would be effective as an agent to increase an AIDS patient's systemic cell-mediated immune defense against HIV by increasing the CD8+ cell count. In the absence of effective treatments, DNCB provided hope to some patients and their physicians; moreover, it was inexpensive and easy to obtain, especially through the many guerrilla clinics that existed at the time.

DNR: *See* DO NOT RESUSCITATE ORDER.

do not resuscitate order (DNR): Instruction given by a patient or family member not to administer cardiopulmonary resuscitation pending the apparent cessation of life. *See also* LIVING WILL and NO CODE.

Dolene: *See* PROPOXYPHENE.

Dolophine: *See* METHADONE.

domestic abuse: Physical, verbal, or emotional violence that occurs between partners or spouses, usually within the home.

double therapy: Concurrent use of two drugs to treat an ailment.

double-blind: A clinical trial or experimental procedure in which neither the subject nor the researcher knows which treatment (drug or placebo) subjects are receiving.

doxil: A liposomal version of the anticancer drug doxorubicin. Used for treating Kaposi's sarcoma.

doxorubicin: A wide-spectrum, antineoplastic, antibiotic agent.

DPT vaccine: A vaccine used for diphtheria, pertussis, and tetanus.

drag queen: A male homosexual who dresses in women's clothing, especially for the purpose of providing public or theatrical entertaining. *See also* TRANSVESTITE.

drama therapy: Use of role play and dramatic improvisation as an adjunct to understanding and coping with difficult life experiences.

dronabinol: Synthetic tetrahydrocannabinol, the psychoactive substance in marijuana. It is used as an antiemetic. Trade names include Deltanyne and Marinol.

droperidol: A drug used for premedication for surgery. Trade name is Inapsine.

drug abuse: The use or overuse of a drug, generally self-administered, in a manner other than that for which it is prescribed.

drug approval: Complex process by which therapeutic agents are certified safe and effective for human use if prescribed and taken according to directions. In the United States, the Food and Drug Administration is responsible for approving all such substances. *See also* CLINICAL TRIAL.

drug culture: Patterns of behavior, thought, and action engendered by individuals' illicit use of controlled substances.

drug development: Process of producing a therapeutic agent ranging from a period of basic scientific research, through research and development, clinical trials, and eventual approval by the Food and Drug Administration (FDA) so that it can be dispensed to patients. Estimated to take an average of 10 years from start to finish, though computer modeling of drug products and a streamlined approval process through the FDA have shortened the time somewhat.

Drug Enforcement Administration: The Drug Enforcement Administration of the Department of Justice is charged with enforcing all controlled substances laws and regulations of the United States. It is the lead agency responsible at the federal level for the development of drug enforcement strategy, programs, planning, and evaluation. Drug Enforcement Administration, Information Services Section (CPI), 700 Army-Navy Drive, Arlington, VA 22202. Telephone: (202) 307-1000. Web site, <http://www.usdoj.gov/dea/>

drug eruption: Inflammation of the skin characterized by itching, redness, and various skin lesions caused by medication. *Also called* DERMATITIS MEDICAMENTOSA.

drug therapy: Treatment of a condition or disease with a pharmaceutical agent or combination of such agents.

DSPN: *See* DISTAL SYMMETRIC POLYNEUROPATHY.

durable power of attorney: A statement declaring a proxy to administer an individual's wishes in the event of incapacity. Durable powers of attorney are not recognized in every state. *See also* DURABLE POWER OF ATTORNEY FOR HEALTH CARE, MEDICAL DIRECTIVE, LIVING WILL, and NO CODE.

durable power of attorney for health care: A document that nominates a proxy to make health care decisions in the event of incapacity. *See also* DURABLE POWER OF ATTORNEY.

Duragesic: *See* FENTANYL TRANSDERMAL SYSTEM.

dying trajectory: A graphical representation of the dying process. Time is recorded along the horizontal axis and nearness to death along the vertical axis. The condition of the dying individual is plotted across time, with the resulting curve being the dying trajectory.

dyke: *See* LESBIAN.

dysfunction: (1) Abnormal, disturbed, impaired, or inadequate functioning of an organ. (2) Abnormal, disturbed, impaired, or inadequate functioning of a social structure (e.g., family).

dysmenorrhea: Pain during menstrual periods.

dysphagia: Difficulty in swallowing, or the inability to swallow.

dyspnea: Difficult or labored breathing; shortness of breath. Dyspnea is sometimes accompanied by pain.

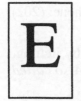

EAP: *See* EMPLOYEE ASSISTANCE PROGRAMS.

early intervention: Refers to instituting anti-HIV therapy early in the course of infection with the hope of driving viral load to undetectable levels, thereby prolonging health.

eating disorders: Mental illness characterized by unhealthy, often life-threatening approaches to the intake of food.

Ebola fever: An acute condition (named for its first known victim in 1976, who came from a village near the Ebola River in Africa) frequently aggravated by hemorrhagic complications and is usually fatal.

EBV: *See* EPSTEIN-BARR VIRUS.

echinacea: Medicianal herb *(Echinacea angust.folia),* a perennial of the daisy family. Some studies suggest a therapeutic and prophylactic effect against upper respiratory allergy symptoms.

echocardiography: (1) A noninvasive technique for examining the internal structure of the heart. (2) A noninvasive diagnostic method that uses the echoes obtained by directing beams of ultrasonic waves through the chest wall to visualize and graphically record internal cardiac structures. *Also called* ULTRASONIC CARDIOGRAPHY.

ecthyma: An ulcerative inflammation of the skin caused by infection, and marked by lesions with crusts or scabs. Variable scarring and pigmentation may result.

edema: A local or generalized condition characterized by excessively large amounts of fluid in the body tissues.

Education and Training Center (ETC): Any one of a group of geographic-specific sites funded by the Health Resources and Services Administration to provide education to health care professionals concerning the acquired immunodeficiency syndrome.

EEG: *See* ELECTROENCEPHALOGRAM.

efavirenz: A non-nucleoside reverse transcriptase inhibitor effective against HIV. Formerly called DMP 266. The trade name is Sustiva.

efficacy: The power or ability to produce intended effects or results.

EIA: *See* ENZYME IMMUNOASSAY.

ejaculation: The expulsion of semen from the male urethra at the peak of sexual excitement.

Elavil: *See* AMITRIPTYLINE.

elderly: (1) Past middle age. (2) Aged.

electroencephalogram (EEG): A recording of the electrical activity of the brain by placing electrodes at various locations on the scalp in order to measure the electrical potential. A technique proven useful as a diagnostic tool in studying convulsive disorders (e.g., epilepsy) and in locating cerebral lesions.

electrolyte: (1) A substance that conducts an electric current and is decomposed by the passage of an electric current in solution (e.g., acids, bases, salts). (2) Ionized salts in blood, tissue, fluids, and cells including chloride, sodium, and potassium.

electrolyte abnormality: A deviation from the normal condition in electrolytes.

electromagnetic field: Field of force created by electric charge in motion. Both electronic and magnetic constituents compose the field. Use of the fields for medically therapeutic purposes is considered an alternative medical practice.

electronic bulletin boards: Early form of electronic communication through computer networks. For the first several years of the AIDS epidemic, activists and patients created many of these systems and established an underground network that spread word about potential therapies, drug availability, and political information.

electrostimulation: Use of electric current to stimulate tissue, such as bone or muscle.

elephant leg: *See* ELEPHANTIASIS.

elephantiasis: (1) A chronic disease characterized by enlargement of certain body parts (especially the legs and genitals), and by the ulceration and hardening of the surrounding skin. (2) A chronic condition caused by inflammation and obstruction of the lymphatic vessels characterized by pronounced hypertrophy (growth due to increase in size of constituent cells) of the skin and subcutaneous tissues. The disease most frequently affects the lower extremities and scrotum. *Also called* BARBADOS LEG, ELEPHANT LEG, and PACHYDERMATOSIS.

ELISA: *See* ENZYME-LINKED IMMUNOSORBENT ASSAY.

embalming: Practice of treating a corpse with preservatives to prevent decay. Existing bodily fluids are extracted from the corpse, and preservatives are added. The practice of embalming is risky for morticians because HIV can be transmitted if universal precautions are not observed.

emergency food services: Programs that provide food and essential household items to AIDS patients who cannot procure such items for themselves.

employee assistance programs (EAP): Programs that exist in the workplace to provide support, referral, and counseling services to employees with problems ranging from alcoholism to bereavement.

Employment and Training Administration (ETA): An office of the Department of Labor, ETA cooperates with state and local workforce development systems to provide high-quality job training, employment, and related services to both workers and employers. U.S. Department of Labor, ETA Office of Public Affairs, 200 Constitution Avenue, N.W., Room N-4700, Washington, DC 20210. Telephone: (202) 219-6871. E-mail is available directly from the Web site, <http://www.doleta.gov/>.

Employment Litigation Section: A section of the Civil Rights Division, Department of Justice, the Employment Litigation Section enforces all federal laws that prohibit discriminatory employment practices on grounds of race, sex, religion, and national origin. Employment Litigation Section of the Civil Rights Division, Department of Justice, P.O. Box 65968, Washington, DC 20035-5968. Telephone: (202) 514-3831; Fax: (202) 514-1105; TDD: (800) 578-5404; Web site, <http://www.usdoj.gov/crt.crt-home.html>.

encephalitis: Inflammation of the brain.

encephalopathy: Any abnormality of cognitive function.

endemic: Native to a particular population or geographic area.

endocarditis: Inflammation of the lining membrane of the heart (endocardium). It may be due to infection occurring as a primary disorder, or in association with another disease. It is usually confined to a heart valve, but, sometimes affects the lining membrane of the cardiac chambers.

Endocet: *See* OXYCODONE.

endocrine abnormality: Any deviation in hormonal secretions.

endocrinology: Study of the body system of glands (e.g., the thyroid) that secrete hormones directly into the bloodstream.

endoscope: An instrument consisting of a tube and optical system for visually examining the inside of a hollow organ or cavity.

endoscopic: Performed by means of an endoscope; pertaining to endoscopy.

endoscopy: Visual inspection of body organs or cavities by means of an endoscope.

enema: (1) The injection of solution into the rectum for the purpose of stimulating bowel activity. (2) The introduction of solution for therapeutic or nutritive purposes. (3) The introduction of fluid to aid in roentgenography. (4) A solution introduced into the rectum.

enteric disease: Any pathological condition involving the small intestine.

enteric pathogen: Any microorganism or substance that is capable of producing a disease in the small intestine.

enteritis: Inflammation of the intestine (especially the small intestine).

env: A gene of HIV that codes for gp160, the precursor of the envelope proteins gp120 and gp41.

envelope gene: The gene that encodes the major virion surface envelope glycoprotein (for the human immunodeficiency virus, this glycoprotein is gp160), and is then processed to form a transmembrane segment (gp41) and a glycosylated external segment (gp120). *See also* ENVELOPE GLYCOPROTEIN and GLYCOPROTEIN.

envelope glycoprotein: The glycosylated external segment (gp120) of the human immunodeficiency virus. The envelope glycoprotein is the major target for the HIV-neutralizing antibody. *See also* GLYCO-PROTEIN.

enzyme immunoassay (EIA): Any of several methods for measuring the protein and protein-bound molecules concerned with the reaction of an antigen with its specific antibody, by using an enzyme covalently linked to an antigen or antibody as a label. The two most common are enzyme-linked immunosorbent assay (ELISA) and enzyme multiplied immunoassay technique (EMIT).

enzyme-linked immunosorbent assay (ELISA): Any enzyme immunoassay method in which an enzyme-labeled immunoreactant (antibody or antigen) and an immunosorbent (antibody or antigen bound to a solid support) are used to detect the presence of specific antibodies or antigens. These assays are more sensitive and simple than radioimmune assay tests, and do not require the use of radioisotopes and an expensive counting device. The ELISA is not completely reliable in detecting the presence of antibodies to the human immunodeficiency virus, making it is necessary to confirm the results using another test such as the Western blot. *See also* ENZYME IMMUNOASSAY.

eosinophil: A cell, histologic element, or structure readily stained with eosin (a synthetic dye used to stain tissues for microscopic examination). Used especially in reference to a granular leukocyte.

eosinophilic: (1) Readily stainable with eosin. (2) Pertaining to eosinophils. *See* EOSINOPHIL.

epidemic: The sudden outbreak and rapid spread of an infectious disease among many people within the same geographical area. Also applied to diseases, injuries, or other events which endanger public health.

epidemic hemorrhagic fever: *See* HANTAVIRUS.

epidemiology: The science concerned with defining and explaining the interrelationships of the factors determining disease frequency and distribution. Studies are generally undertaken to establish programs for the prevention and control of disease development and spread of disease.

epistaxis: Hemorrhage from the nose; a nosebleed.

epithelial cell: An irregularly-shaped cell that has a single nucleus. Frequently, two or three are joined together.

epithelium: The purely cellular, nonvascular layer covering the free surfaces of the body (cutaneous, mucous, and serous).

Epivir: *See* LAMIVUDINE.

Epogen: *See* ERYTHROPOIETIN.

Epstein-Barr virus (EBV): A herpes-like virus, discovered in 1964, that is the causative agent in infectious mononucleosis. It is also associated with Burkitt's lymphoma and nasopharyngeal carcinoma.

Equal Employment Opportunity Commission (EEOC): The EEOC strives to promote equal opportunity in employment through administrative and judicial enforcement of federal civil rights laws, and through education and technical assistance. Complete field office contact information and e-mail is available online through the EEOC Web site. Equal Employment Opportunity Commission, L Street, N.W., Washington, DC 20507. Telephone: (800) 669-4000 (bilingual English/Spanish); TDD: (800) 669-6820.

erotica: Materials pertaining to sexual desire or passion.

eroticism: Sexual desire.

erythema multiforme: A macular eruption with dark red papules or tubercles. Usually found on extremities and appearing in successive eruptions of short duration. May appear in separate rings, concentric rings, patches, distributed elevations, and patterned arrangements. Not associated with itching or burning.

Erythrocin: *See* ERYTHROMYCIN.

erythrocyte: (1) A circulating red blood cell. (2) A mature red blood cell or corpuscle shaped in the form of a nonnucleated, yellowish, biconcave disk. It consists of a respiratory pigment (hemoglobin), enclosed in a membrane of proteins and lipoid substances.

By the nature of its composition, the erythrocyte is adapted to transport oxygen throughout the body. *Also called* RED BLOOD CELL or RED BLOOD CORPUSCLE.

erythrocyte aggregation: Collection of red blood cells probably resulting from changes in the negative surface charge of the cells caused by the dielectric effect of proteins in the surrounding plasma.

erythrocyte count: A count of the number of red blood cells per unit volume in a sample of venous blood.

erythrocyte sedimentation rate (ESR): The rate at which erythrocytes (the circulating red blood cells) settle from a well-mixed specimen of blood. The venous blood is placed in a long, narrow tube, and the distance the top of the column of red cells falls in a specified time interval under specific conditions is the rate. The rate at which the cells sediment depends upon the size of the clumps into which the erythrocytes aggregate, and the size of the clumps depends upon the amount of plasma proteins (especially fibrinogen and immunoglobulins). The ESR is an indicator of inflammatory disease and other conditions in which it (the rate) is usually elevated.

erythrocytophagy: The consumption or engulfment of erythrocytes by other cells (e.g., erythrocytes consumed by histiocytes of the reticuloendothelial system).

erythromycin: An antibiotic produced by *Streptomyces erythreus,* which appears as a yellowish, crystalline powder. Administered orally, it is effective against many gram-positive and certain gram-negative bacteria. It may also be applied topically in the treatment of certain infections. Used to treat patients who are allergic to penicillin, and in the treatment of penicillin-resistant infections. The trade name is ERYTHROCIN.

erythrophagocytosis: *See* ERYTHROCYTOPHAGY.

erythropoietin: Glycoprotein hormone, secreted chiefly by the kidney in the adult and the liver in the fetus, that acts on erythroid stem cells of the bone marrow to stimulate differentiation and proliferation. The trade name is Procrit.

esophagitis: Inflammation of the esophagus.

esophagoscope: A flexible or rigid instrument, equipped with an optical system, inserted into the esophagus for diagnostic and therapeutic purposes (obtaining specimens or removing foreign substances).

esophagoscopy: An endoscopic examination of the esophagus using an esophagoscope.

Esophotrast: *See* BARIUM SULFATE.

ESR: *See* ERYTHROCYTE SEDIMENTATION RATE.

estate planning: To form a plan concerning the dispensation of property and possessions upon death.

ETC: *See* EDUCATION AND TRAINING CENTER.

etiology: The study of the cause or origin of a disease; the cause or origin of a disease.

etoposide: (1) An antineoplastic. (2) A semisynthetic derivative of podophyllotoxin, administered intravenously, and used to prevent the development, growth, or proliferation of malignant cells.

eucalyptus: Any of a group of mostly Australian evergreen trees. Used as a cough suppressant and an expectorant. The volatile oil obtained from eucalyptus is combined with a sugar base to form lozenges which suppress coughs, apparently by stimulating saliva production and secretion. The volatile oil is also used in balms and ointments, nasal sprays and inhalers, and mouthwashes. Eucalyptus leaves may be prepared as a tea that is an effective cough remedy.

eustachian dysfunction: Abnormal or impaired functioning of the auditory tube (eustachian tube), which extends from the middle ear to the pharynx. When the passage is blocked, otitis media may develop.

euthanasia: The act of willfully ending life in individuals who have an incurable disease.

exanthema: *See* ACUTE HIV EXANTHEM.

Expanded Access: A program that allows persons who meet certain criteria but are not enrolled in a clinical trial to receive an experimental drug. The administering physician monitors the person's response to the drug, and reports these results to the pharmaceutical company that manufactures the experimental drug. The existence of this program is due mainly to the pressure applied by AIDS activists for reform within the drug approval process.

extended care organizations: Any of a group of organizations or institutions providing medical care for patients who require long-term custodial or medical care, especially for a chronic disease or one requiring prolonged rehabilitation therapy.

extrahepatic disease: A pathological condition occurring outside the liver.

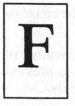

facial nerve paralysis: Paralysis affecting the muscles of the face in which the seventh cranial nerve is involved.

factor: (1) Any substance or activity required to produce a result. (2) A contributing cause in an action. (3) A gene (hereditary factor).

factor VIII: (1) Blood coagulation factor. (2) An antihemophilic factor participating only in the intrinsic pathway of blood coagulation. Deficiency of this factor, when transmitted as a sex-linked recessive trait, causes classic hemophilia. *Also called* ANTIHEMOPHILIC GLOBULIN (AHG) and ANTIHEMOPHILIC FACTOR A.

Fair Housing Amendments Act: Amended numerous times in the 1970s and 1980s, the Act is an outgrowth of the Federal Housing Act of 1968. Designed to ban housing discrimination based on disability, and covers most real estate transactions (financing, rental, sale); the Act provides limited exemptions for religious organizations and private clubs as well as owners of fewer than 3 units who do not use real estate agents, and owner-occupied buildings with fewer than 4 units.

false-negative: (1) A test result incorrectly denoting the absence of the abnormality or disease for which the test is administered. (2) An individual whose test result incorrectly excludes him or her from a diagnostic category.

false-positive: (1) A test result incorrectly denoting the presence of the abnormality or disease for which the test is administered. (2) An individual whose test result incorrectly assigns him or her to a diagnostic category.

famciclovir: A systemic antiviral drug shown to be effective in treating herpes zoster and postherpetic neuralgia.

family: (1) A group of people related by ancestry or marriage. (2) A group of people living in the same household. (3) A group of people considering themselves related by a common bond. (4) In biological classification, a category of plants and animals between an order and a genus.

family planning: Use of various contraceptive devices or strategies to space or limit the number of children born to a union.

family practice: Comprehensive medical care with particular emphasis on the family unit in which the physician's continuing responsibility for health care is not limited by the patient's age, sex, disease entity, or organ system involved.

Famvir: *See* FAMCICLOVIR.

fatigue: (1) A feeling of tiredness or weariness. (2) A decrease in efficiency or reduction in response to stimulation. Fatigue generally results from continued exertion or overactivity, but many HIV-related infections result in fatigue with little or no effort.

FDA: *See* FOOD AND DRUG ADMINISTRATION.

fear: (1) A feeling of anxiety and agitation caused by the close proximity of danger, evil, pain, etc. (2) A feeling of uneasiness or concern. (3) Fright; dread.

feces: (1) The excrement consisting of food residue, bacteria, mucus, and exfoliated cells discharged from the intestines by way of the anus. (2) Body waste.

Federal Bureau of Investigation (FBI): The FBI is the primary investigative branch of the United States Department of Justice. It has the authority and responsibility to investigate all crimes assigned to it as well as to provide law enforcement agencies throughout the United States with cooperative services such as training of law enforcement personnel and forensic laboratory work. Federal Bureau of Investigation, J. Edgar Hoover Building, 935 Pennsylvania Avenue, N.W.,

Washington, DC 20353. Telephone: (202) 324-3000; Web site, <http://www.fbi.gov/contact.htm>. Direct links to all FBI field offices throughout the United States are available from this Web site, with complete contact information provided.

Federal Mediation and Conciliation Services: Created by Congress in 1947, this is an independent agency that promotes sound, stable labor-management relations including those involving health and benefit issues. Federal Mediation and Conciliation Services, 2100 K Street, N.W., Washington, DC 29427. Telephone: (202) 606-8100; Fax: (202) 606-4216. E-mail is available directly from the Web site, <http://www.fmcs.gov/>.

Federal Rehabilitation Act: Enacted in 1973, its purpose is to ban discrimination by any federal agency and any institution receiving federal financial assistance.

Federal Trade Commission (FTC): Established in 1914, the FTC is responsible for consumer protection in many areas including investments, products and services, credit, diet, health, and fitness. A complaint form and e-mail are available directly from the Web site, <http://www.ftc.gov>. Federal Trade Commission, CRC-240, Washington, DC 20580. Telephone: (202) 326-2000.

fellatio: Oral stimulation of the penis.

female condom: A soft, loose-fitting polyurethane sheath, closed at one end, with flexible rings at both. The device is inserted into the vagina by compressing the inner ring and pushing it in. Properly positioned, the ring at the closed end covers the cervix, and the sheath lines the walls of the vagina. The outer ring remains outside the vagina, covering the labia. *See also* CONDOM.

female-to-female transmission: (1) Sexual transmission of a communicable disease from one female to another female. (2) The passage or transfer of any pathological condition from a female to another female.

female-to-male transmission: (1) Sexual transmission of a communicable disease from a female to a male. (2) The passage or transfer of any pathological condition from a female to a male.

feminism: (1) The theory of the economic, political, and social equality of the sexes. (2) Organized activities on behalf of women's rights and interests.

fentanyl patch: *See* FENTANYL TRANSDERMAL SYSTEM.

fentanyl transdermal system: A potent narcotic analgesic, applied to the skin using a patch, administered to manage or relieve pain. The trade name is Duragesic.

fetus: The unborn offspring of a human, or an animal, while in the uterus or within an egg during the latter stages of development. In humans, this period is considered to be 2 to 3 months after conception until birth. Prior to this period, the fertilized egg is called an embryo.

fever: Elevation of body temperature above normal; hyperpyrexia. The normal body temperature taken orally is 98.6°F. This may vary 1° above or 2° below normal and can still be considered in the normal range. Normal rectal temperatures are 0.5° to 1.0° higher than oral temperatures.

fibrocyst: A fibrous tumor that has undergone cystic degeneration or one that has accumulated fluid in the interspaces.

fibrocystic disease of the breast: A chronic disorder comprising 3 variants, which range from lesions consisting primarily of an overgrowth of fibrous tissue to those characterized by dominance of the proliferation of the epithelial parenchyma, to a form of dysplasia characterized by both stromal and epithelial hyperplasia with the formation of cysts.

FIC: *See* FOGARTY INTERNATIONAL CENTER.

Filoviridae: A family of viruses containing filamentous virions. There is one genus known as filovirus.

filovirus: A genus of the family Filoviridae containing two species; Ebola virus and Marburg virus. Both were originally associated with African monkeys but are capable of causing severe hemorrhagic diseases in humans. Transmission is by close personal contact.

financial assistance services: Any of a group of social service programs in which financial aid is provided to those in need.

fingering: *See* DIGITAL INTERCOURSE.

first aid: Immediate intervention following an accident or injury to alleviate complications such as shock or blood loss.

fist fucking: *See* BRACHIOPROCTIC EROTICISM.

fisting: *See* BRACHIOPROCTIC EROTICISM.

Fluax: *See* INFLUENZA VIRUS VACCINE.

fluconazole: An antifungal drug approved by the Food and Drug Administration for the treatment of cryptococcal meningitis, and oral and esophogeal candidiasis. The trade name is Diflucan.

flucytosine: An antifungal drug, appearing as a whitish, crystalline powder, administered orally to treat yeast and fungal infections (such as those caused by *Candida* and/or *Cryptococcus*-like endocarditis, septicemia, or urinary tract infections). The trade name is Ancobon.

Fluogen: *See* INFLUENZA VIRUS VACCINE.

fluoxetine: The first highly specific serotonin uptake inhibitor. It is used as an antidepressant and often has a more acceptable side-effects profile than traditional antidepressants. Trade name is Prozac.

fluphenazine: A drug used in the treatment of psychoses. The trade name is Prolixin.

Fogarty International Center (FIC): As part of the National Institute of Health, the Center is dedicated to advancing the health of the people of the United States and other nations through international scientific cooperation. In pursuit of its mission, the Fogarty International Center fosters biomedical research partnerships between U.S. scientists and foreign counterparts through grants, fellowships, and international agreements, and provides leadership in international scientific policy and research strategies.Fogarty International Center, 9000 Rockville Pike, Bethesda, MD 20892. Public Affairs Office: (301) 496-2075, Director's Office: (301) 496-1415. E-mail is available directly from the Web site, <http://www.nih.gov/fic/>.

folic acid: A member of the vitamin B complex necessary for various metabolic reactions, and used in the treatment of sprue. Inadequate amounts of folic acid cause megaloblastic anemia. Folic acid is found naturally in green plants, liver, and yeast. *Also called* LACTOBACILLUS CASEI FACTOR, LIVER LACTOBACILLUS CASEI FACTOR, PTEROYLMONOGLUTAMIC ACID, and VITAMIN M. The trade name is Folvite.

folinic acid: A derivative of folic acid used to counteract the effects of folic acid antagonists, and in treating anemia caused by a deficiency of folic acid. The trade name is Calcium Folinate. *Also called* CITROVORUM FACTOR and LEUCOVORIN.

follicle: A small sac or cavity for excretion or secretion.

folliculitis: Inflammation of a follicle or follicles.

Folvite: *See* FOLIC ACID.

fomivirsen: First antisense drug to be reviewed by the Food and Drug Administration, fomivirsen works at the genetic level to block the production of proteins that cause disease. It was approved August 27, 1998. Fomivirsen slows the progression of cytomegalovirus retinitis, an aggressive disease that formerly left many AIDS patients blind. The trade name is Vitravene.

fomivirsen sodium: Drug used to treat cytomegalovirus retinitis. It is injected directly into the eye.

Food and Drug Administration (FDA): Founded in 1931 under the Agriculture Appropriation Act, it is charged with protecting the Nation against impure and unsafe foods, cosmetics, drugs, and other potential hazards. Prior to January 1, 1907, when the 1906 Food and Drug Act became effective, the goals of the organization were carried out under similar law enforcement functions in existence under various organizational titles. Food and Drug Administration, Department of Health and Human Services, Public Health Service, 5600 Fishers Lane, Rockville, MD 20857. Telephone: (888) 463-6332. E-mail is available directly from the Web site, <http://www.fda.gov/>.

food service industry: The segment of the profit sector of the economy concerned with the production, preparation, and presentation of food.

Food Stamp Program (FSP): Operated through the Food and Nutrition Service of the Department of Agriculture, the FSP is designed to serve as the first line of defense against hunger in the

United States. The program theoretically enables low-income families and individuals to purchase nutritious food with coupons and Electronic Benefits Transfer cards. Food Stamp Program, United States Department of Agriculture, 14th and Independence, S.W., Washington, DC 20250. Telephone: (800) 221-5689. E-mail and hotline numbers in each state are easily accessible via the FSP Web site, <http://www.fns.usda.gov/fsp/>.

Fortovase: *See* SAQUINAVIR.

foscarnet: An antiviral drug approved by the Food and Drug Administration for the treatment of cytomegalovirus retinitis. The trade name is FOSCAVIR. *Also called* TRISODIUM PHOSPHONOFORMATE, TRISODIUM CARBOXY PHOSPHATE, and PHOSPHONOFORMIC ACID TRISODIUM SALT.

Foscavir: *See* FOSCARNET.

foster care: Affording, providing, or receiving parental care though not related by blood or legal ties.

Foundation of Pharmacists and Corporate America for AIDS Education: Founded in 1988, this organization consists of associations, corporations, pharmacies, and individuals that seek to support pharmacists who provide education and outreach programs designed to prevent the spread of HIV and AIDS. Foundation of Pharmacists and Corporate America for AIDS Education, 700 Fifth Street N.W., Suite 303, Washington, DC 20001. Telephone: (202) 371-1830.

"Four-H Club": A term applied by American epidemiologists in the early years of the epidemic to high-risk populations. This term was used in the early 1980s, prior to current AIDS nomenclature, and at a time when it was unsure as to how best to portray those individuals affected by the epidemic. The term included Haitians, homosexuals, heroin addicts, and hemophiliacs, but was expanded by some also to include hookers. It is now considered inappropriate because it perpetuates the stigma associated with HIV and AIDS by characterizing high-risk populations as deserving of infection based on behavior.

fraud: Misconduct involving deception.

freebase: A form of cocaine in which the hydrochloride salt is alkalinized, extracted with an organic solvent (e.g., ether), and then heated. After inhalation, the drug is absorbed rapidly through the lungs.

freebasing: The inhalation of a form of cocaine known as freebase.

French kiss: (1) A passionate kiss with the lips parted and tongues touching. (2) To kiss passionately with the lips parted and tongues touching.

frottage: Passionate rubbing between partners, clothed or unclothed, for the purpose of sexual stimulation. Sometimes taught as a safe sex technique. *Also called* PRINCETON RUB.

fungal encephalitis: Inflammation of the brain resulting from invasion by a pathogenic fungus.

fungal infection: The state or condition in which the body, or a part of it, is invaded by a pathogenic fungus.

fungi: Plural of fungus.

fungicidin: *See* NYSTATIN.

fungus: A general term used to denote a group of vegetable cellular organisms, which are characterized by the absence of chlorophyll. They exist on organic matter and are generally simple in structure and form. Included in this group are molds, yeasts, rusts, and mushrooms.

furuncle: A painful, deep-seated nodule formed in the skin by circumscribed inflammation, enclosing a central core. It is caused by staphylococci, which enter through the hair follicles. Formation is promoted by local irritation and digestive derangement. It usually ends in pus formation and necrosis. *Also called* BOIL and FURUNCULUS.

furunculosis: The persistent simultaneous occurrence of furuncles.

furunculus: *See* FURUNCLE.

fusion inhibitors: A drug that inhibits the binding of HIV's envelope to a host cell's receptors.

gag gene: The gene which encodes the major internal viral structural proteins of the human immunodeficiency virus (p17, p24, p15).

ganciclovir: (1) A drug used to treat cytomegalovirus retinitis. (2) An acyclic nucleoside structurally related to acyclovir, and an effective antiviral against cytomegalovirus (CMV) in vitro. The drug has been carefully studied only in the treatment of cytomegalovirus retinitis, and has been shown to halt retinal destruction during administration. When administration is withdrawn, disease progression resumes. Licensed by the Food and Drug Administration in 1989 for treating sight-threatening cytomegalovirus retinitis, its use for treatment of other CMV diseases is still considered investigational. Formerly called DHPG or dihydroxypropoxymethyl. The trade name is Cytovene.

ganglion: (1) A collection of nerve cell bodies located outside of the central nervous system. (2) A benign cystic tumor developing on a tendon or aponeurosis, sometimes occurring in the back of the wrist or dorsum of the foot. (3) A knot-like mass.

garlic: An herb related to the lillies and grown for its pungent bulbs used in cooking. Also used as a traditional remedy. It contains allicin, the pungent active ingredient, which may reduce blood cholesterol and inhibit platelet aggregation.

gastric anacidity: *See* ACHLORHYDRIA.

gastroenterology: A branch of medicine dealing with the alimentary canal.

gastrointestinal dysfunction: Abnormal, impaired, or inadequate functioning of the stomach and intestines.

gastrointestinal tract: The stomach and intestines.

gay: Generally refers to male homosexuals, but may include homosexual women as well. The term has political, psychological, and social implications that stretch beyond the realm of sexual orientation. *See also* HOMOSEXUAL and LESBIAN.

gay bowel syndrome: A general term used to denote a constellation of intestinal diseases among gay men including proctitis, proctocolitis, and enteritis. The term was widely used in the 1970s with the dramatic increase in enteric diseases within the gay community thought to be directly linked to anal intercourse.

gay lymph node syndrome: A term applied to generalized lymphadenopathy (with benign reactive changes shown in biopsy) prior to 1981 when the Centers for Disease Control published the first description of persistent generalized lymphadenopathy.

Gay Men's Health Crisis (GMHC): Founded in 1982 as a social service agency for the clinical treatment of the acquired immunodeficiency syndrome. It provides a variety of services (therapy, education, recreation services, crisis counseling, a buddy program, and advocacy) to AIDS patients and their families. GMHC also maintains a hotline, speakers' bureau, and library. It sponsors AIDS education programs and compiles statistics. Gay Men's Health Crisis, 19 W. 24th Street, New York, NY 10011. Telephone: (212) 807-6664.

gay plague: Since gay men were the first infected and continue to constitute the greatest number of reported cases in the United States, this term was often used to denote the acquired immunodeficiency syndrome, particularly in the early years of the epidemic.

gay pneumonia: Initially used to denote *Pneumocystis carinii* pneumonia.

gaybashing: Abuse, injury, or death motivated by bias based on homosexual sexual orientation.

gay-related immune deficiency (GRID): One of a group of names initially used to denote the acquired immunodeficiency syndrome. The current nomenclature was adopted in 1981. *See also* ACQUIRED COMMUNITY IMMUNE DEFICIENCY SYNDROME, COMMUNITY ACQUIRED IMMUNE DEFICIENCY SYNDROME, and ACQUIRED IMMUNODEFICIENCY SYNDROME.

GCSF: *See* GRANULOCYTE COLONY-STIMULATING FACTOR.

gene: The basic biological unit of heredity. They are self-producing, ultramicroscopic structures, which are transmitted from parent to offspring. Each gene is a segment on a DNA molecule that stores the information necessary for the transcription of information by RNA and synthesis of proteins, and occupies a specific location on a chromosome. Hereditary traits are dependent on the pairing of genes in the same position on a pair of chromosomes.

gene amplification: A selective increase in the number of copies of a gene coding for specific protein without a proportional increase in other genes.

gene therapy: The introduction of new genes into cells for the purpose of treating disease by restoring or adding gene expression.

general internal medicine: The branch of medicine that treats diseases of the internal organs by other than surgical means.

genetic engineering: Directed modification of the gene complement of a living organism by such techniques as altering the DNA, substituting genetic material by means of a virus, transplanting whole nuclei, transplanting cell hybrids, etc.

genetic expression: The phenotypic manifestation of a gene or genes by the processes of gene action.

genetic research: The study and examination of reproduction, heredity, and its variance.

genetics: A branch of biology dealing with heredity and variation.

genital herpes simplex: Herpes simplex located in the inguinal area.

genital self-examination (GSE): The inspection of one's own genitals, usually for signs of disease.

genital wart: (1) A small, tumorous growth on the skin of the genitalia caused by a virus. (2) A circumscribed epidermal lesion of the genitalia with a horny surface caused by a human papillomavirus.

genitalia: The various internal and external organs related to reproduction.

genus: In biology, the taxonomic division between the species and the family.

Giardia: A genus of flagellate protozoa, usually nonpathogenic. They inhabit the small intestine in humans, and are characterized by the presence of a large sucking disk on the ventral body surface (the means by which the organism attaches itself to the intestinal epithelium).

Giardia intestinalis: See GIARDIA LAMBLIA.

Giardia lamblia: A species of *Giardia* found in humans that may cause giardiasis. They are transmitted by ingestion of fecally contaminated matter, and are found worldwide. *Also called* GIARDIA INTESTINALIS and LAMBLIA INTESTINALIS.

giardiasis: (1) A protozoan infection. (2) A common infection with the flagellate protozoan *Giardia lamblia.* Infection is spread through contaminated food or water. Most cases are asymptomatic. When present, symptoms include anorexia, cramps, diarrhea, fever, nausea, weakness, weight loss, and vomiting. *Also called* LAMBLIASIS.

ginger: The pungent, aromatic rootstock of a tropical plant used especially as a spice and for its medicinal value. This herb is believed to be effective in fighting colds, colitis, digestive disorders, and flu. It is also believed to help increase saliva secretion, assist the circulatory system, and help increase stamina.

ginseng: A Chinese or American herb valued for its aromatic root. Some believe ginseng to be an aphrodisiac or stimulant. In some cultures, it is believed to stimulate RNA and DNA activity in the cells, helping to retard the aging process.

Glaxo Wellcome Inc.: A pharmaceutical company that includes AZT among its products. Glaxo Wellcome Inc., P.O. Box 13398, Research Triangle Park, Durham, NC 27709. Telephone: (919) 248-3000 or (888) TALK 2GW.

Global Programme on AIDS: *See* JOINT UNITED NATIONS PROGRAM ON AIDS.

GLQ-223: A drug derived from the Chinese cucumber, tested in Phase I clinical trials, and shown to be effective against the human immunodeficiency virus in vitro by selectively destroying infected cells.

glutamic acid: A nonessential amino acid believed to improve mental capacities and aid in combating fatigue.

glutamine: An essential component in the chemical breakdown of proteins. Found in the juices of many plants.

glutathione: (1) A combination of amino acids fundamentally important in cellular respiration; takes up and gives off hydrogen. (2) A tripeptide of glutamate, cysteine, and glycine found in small quantities in active animal and plant tissues. It is essential for cellular respiration, and functions in redox reactions such as serving as a cofactor for enzymes and destroying or detoxifying harmful compounds.

glycine: A nonessential amino acid believed to play a role in building and maintaining a strong immune system.

glycoprotein: (1) Any of a class of compounds in which a carbohydrate group is combined with a protein. (2) Any of a class of compounds (this group includes the mucins, the mucoids, and the chondroproteins) consisting of a carbohydrate and a protein. In decomposition, they yield a product frequently capable of reducing alkaline solutions of cupric oxide.

glycyrrhiza: A dried root used as a flavoring agent in compounding medicine. Also used as a demulcent, an expectorant, and a mild laxative.

GMHC: *See* GAY MEN'S HEALTH CRISIS.

golden shower: (1) The act of urinating on an individual for sexual pleasure. (2) Being urinated upon for sexual pleasure. *See also* WATER SPORT and UROLAGNEA.

gonad: (1) A gland or organ that produces reproductive cells in animals. (2) A general term referring to a gamete-producing gland, which includes both the female ovary and male testis.

gonorrhea: (1) An infectious venereal disease. (2) A specific contagious inflammation of the genital mucous membrane of either sex caused by infection due to *Neisseria gonorrhoeae*. Often asymptomatic in females, gonorrhea is characterized by urethritis in males and accompanied by slow, painful urination containing mucous and pus. Other parts of the body (heart, throat, joints, rectum, and skin) may also be affected.

gossypol: A toxic chemical (with antifertility properties in males) that is yellowish in appearance, and found in cotton seed. It is detoxified by heating.

gotu kola: An herb believed to promote memory and help alleviate mental fatigue.

gp41: The transmembrane segment of the human immunodeficiency virus.

gp120: The glycosylated external segment of the human immuno-deficiency virus (envelope glycoprotein).

gp160: The envelope gene of the human immunodeficiency virus.

gram-negative bacteria: Bacteria that, in Gram's method of staining, lose the stain and take the color of the red counterstain. *See* GRAM'S METHOD.

gram-positive bacteria: Bacteria that, in Gram's method of staining, retain the stain. *See* GRAM'S METHOD.

Gram's method: A differential method of staining bacteria in which the specimen is first placed in aniline water-gentian violet or carbolic-gentian violet, rinsed in water and immersed in an iodine solution. It is rinsed in water again and placed in strong alcohol for several minutes, rinsed again, and dipped in a dilute eosin solution. Gram-negative bacteria decolorize and assume the counterstain, while gram-positive bacteria stain a dark violet.

granisetron: A serotonin receptor antagonist that has been used as an antiemetic for cancer chemotherapy patients. The trade name is Kytril.

granulocyte colony-stimulating factor (GCSF): Biological therapy sometimes used to combat the adverse effects resulting from antiretroviral therapies, ganciclovir therapy for cytomegalovirus infections, chemotherapy for AIDS-related cancers, and antibiotic therapies for various opportunistic infections.

granulocyte-macrophage colony-stimulating factor: Biological therapy sometimes used to combat the adverse effects resulting from chemotherapy for AIDS-related lymphoma. Not widely used because of the severity of side effects, especially the possibility that it may stimulate HIV replication.

GRID: *See* GAY-RELATED IMMUNE DEFICIENCY.

grief: The normal emotional response to a recognized loss. A process through which the bereaved pass in order to recover from the loss; it includes emotions similar to those associated with dying such as denial, anger, and acceptance. The grief process is often accompanied by physical manifestations such as a change in sleep patterns, hollow feeling in the chest or abdomen, uncontrollable sighing, and tightness of the throat. Grief is generally self-limited, subsiding in a reasonable amount of time. *See also* BEREAVEMENT and MOURNING.

group psychological treatment models: Any of a variety of psychotherapeutic approaches involving 2 or more patients for the purpose of each patient's mental illness or improving health.

group therapy: A form of simultaneous psychotherapy involving 2 or more patients for the purpose of treating each patient's mental illness or improving health.

group-specific complement: A series of enzymatic proteins in normal serum that, in the presence of a sensitizer specific for a given group, destroy bacteria and other cells. The complement is important in maintaining a normal state of health. *See also* IMMUNITY, ANTIBODY, and ANTIGEN.

GSE: *See* GENITAL SELF-EXAMINATION.

guerilla clinic: Any of a group of for-profit facilities established early in the AIDS epidemic for the purpose of dispensing black-market drugs, or providing treatments or therapies not approved in traditional medical channels. They were similar to back-room abortionists or snake oil salesmen.

guided imagery: The use of mental images produced by the imagination as a form of psychotherapy. It is used in the treatment of mental disorders and in recovery from an infectious disease.

Guillain-Barré syndrome: Polyneuritis with progressive muscular weakness of extremities that may lead to paralysis. Usually occurs after recovery from an infectious disease. It has also occurred after immunization with influenza vaccine.

guilt: A feeling of self-reproach resulting from doing something perceived to be wrong.

gummatous syphilis: Late benign syphilis.

Gyne-Lotrimin: *See* CLOTRIMAZOLE.

gynecological disorder: A disturbance in any of the female reproductive organs including the breasts.

gynecology: A branch of medicine dealing with the diseases and hygiene of women.

gynecomastia: Abnormal enlargement of breast tissue in males. Reported side effect of some antiretroviral therapies.

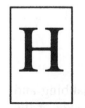

HAART: *See* HIGHLY ACTIVE ANTIRETROVIRAL THERAPY.

hairy leukoplakia (HL): A white lesion generally found on the lateral margins of the tongue. Lesions may vary in size and shape, and have an irregular surface. They may spread to cover the dorsal surface of the tongue and downward on to the ventral surface. Hairy leukoplakia is usually asymptomatic, and is most likely viral induced (Epstein-Barr virus has been associated with HL tissue).

Haitian Coalition on AIDS (HCA): Founded in 1983, this organization is divided into local, state, and regional groups. It seeks to educate the general public concerning AIDS and the Haitian community, promote AIDS education to the Haitian community, and provide services to those members of the community with AIDS and their families. Haitian Coalition on AIDS, 50 Court Street, Suite 110, Brooklyn, NY 11201. Telephone: (718) 855-0972.

Haldol: *See* HALOPERIDOL.

half-life: The amount of time required for one-half of a substance to be eliminated from the living tissue, organ, or organism into which it has been introduced.

haloperidol: An antipsychotic drug used primarily to treat schizophrenia and other psychoses. The trade name is Haldol.

hantavirus: A genus of the family *Bunyaviridae* causing hantavirus infections. It was first identified during the Korean War. Infection is found primarily in rodents and humans. Transmission does not appear to involve arthropods. There are two major clinical manifestations; hemorrhagic fever with renal syndrome, found worldwide in various forms, and hantavirus pulmonary syndrome, found only in the Americas.

Hassal's corpuscles: Oval or spherical bodies present in the medulla of the thymus, consisting of concentrically arranged epithelial cells surrounding a core of degenerated cells.

hate crimes: Illegal acts committed because of prejudice toward a specific ethnic or other distinct group perceived to be different from the "norm."

HBV: *See* HEPATITIS B VIRUS.

HCA: *See* HAITIAN COALITION ON AIDS.

HCFA: *See* HEALTH CARE FINANCING ADMINISTRATION.

HCW: *See* HEALTH CARE WORKER.

headache: Pain, ranging from dull and throbbing to stabbing and severe, localized in an area of the head, especially one side or the other, the back of the head, or the area over an eye. Therapeutic options vary depending on the etiology of the headache and whether it is acute or chronic. As is true of the general population, headaches are a common complaint of HIV-infected individuals at all stages of the infection. They may result from activity of the HIV-1 virus itself, various opportunistic infections, or as an adverse effect of medication.

health behavior: Any behavior expressed by individuals to protect, promote, or maintain their health status. This may include diet, exercise, and lifestyle choices.

health care: The charge of providing for mental and physical well-being.

Health Care Financing Administration (HCFA): A department of the Health and Human Services Operating Division, HCFA administers the Medicare, Medicaid, and Child Health Insurance programs, which together cover some of the medical costs for more than 75 million individuals in the United States. Additionally, HCFA is responsible for the regulation of all laboratory testing, except that involving research performed on human beings, in the United States. Health Care Financing Administration, Information Clearinghouse, 7500 Security Boulevard, Baltimore MD 21244. Telephone: (410) 786-3000; Web site, <http://www.hcfa.gov/>.

health care provider: An individual who furnishes the means by which others obtain mental and physical well-being (e.g., physicians, nurses).

health care reform: Innovation and improvement of the health care system by reappraisal, amendment of services, and removal of faults and abuses in providing and distributing health services to patients.

health care worker (HCW): An individual who is employed in the profession responsible for the provision of mental and physical well-being (e.g., medical professionals, laboratory personnel, technicians, physical facility staff).

health maintenance organization (HMO): Organized systems for providing comprehensive prepaid health care that have five basic attributes: (1) provide care in a defined geographic area; (2) provide or ensure delivery of an agreed-upon set of basic and supplemental health maintenance and treatment services; (3) provide care to a voluntarily enrolled group of persons; (4) require their enrollees to use the services of designated providers; and (5) receive reimbursement through a predetermined, fixed, periodic prepayment made by the enrollee without regard to the degree of services provided.

Health Resources and Services Administration (HRSA): The Administration responsible for leadership within the Public Health Service concerning general health services and resource issues relating to access, cost, equity, and quality of care. To accomplish this goal, it participates in the federal campaign against AIDS by funding service demonstration projects in major cities, establishing centers to train health care professionals concerning AIDS, supporting renovation of health care facilities for AIDS patients, and awarding pediatric health care grants for the care of AIDS babies. Health Resources and Services Administration, Department of Health and Human Services, Public Health Service, 5600 Fishers Lane, Rockville, MD 20857. Telephone: (301) 443-2086. E-mail is available directly from the Web site, <http://www.hrsa.dhhs.gov/>.

heart attack: *See* MYOCARDIAL INFARCTION.

helminthiasis: Having intestinal parasites or worms.

helminthic infestation: The invasion by, and harboring of, parasitic worms that produce injurious effects.

helper cell: Differentiated T lymphocyte whose cooperation is necessary for the production of antibodies against most antigens. Help-

er cells are marked by the T4 antigen in humans. *See also* LYMPHO-
CYTE.

hematocrit: (1) An instrument for separating solids from plasma in
the blood. (2) The volume of erythrocytes packed by centrifugation
in a given volume of blood. The hematocrit is expressed as the
percentage of total blood volume that consists of erythrocytes, or as
the volume in cubic centimeters of erythrocytes packed by centrifugation of blood.

hematologic abnormality: A deviation from the norm in the blood
or blood-forming tissues.

hematologic disorder: Pathological condition of the blood or
blood-forming tissues.

hematologic test: Any method used to determine abnormalities in
the blood or blood-forming tissues.

hematology: The science related to blood and the blood-forming
tissues.

hemodialysis: A method for artificially performing the function of
the kidneys (in removing wastes or toxins from the blood) by circulating the blood through a series of tubes made of semipermeable
membranes, which are bathed in solutions that selectively remove
undesirable elements.

hemodialyzer: An apparatus used in performing hemodialysis.

hemoglobin: (1) The oxygen-carrying pigment of the red blood
cells. (2) The iron-containing pigment of the erythrocytes. It is
formed by the developing erythrocyte in bone marrow, and serves
to transport oxygen from the lungs to the tissues.

hemophilia: A hereditary blood disease characterized by prolonged
coagulation time. The blood fails to clot and hemorrhage occurs.
Although transmitted by the female who carries the recessive gene,
hemophilia occurs almost exclusively in males. There are two main
forms: hemophilia A (classic hemophilia) resulting from factor VIII
deficiency, and hemophilia B, resulting from factor IX deficiency.

hemophiliac: An individual exhibiting hemophilia.

hemorrhage: The abnormal discharge of blood from the vessels. It
may be arterial, capillary, or venous from blood vessels into tissues

or into or from the body. Hemorrhages are classified according to size: petechiae is very small; purpura measures up to 1 centimeter; ecchymoses is larger than 1 centimeter.

hemorrhagic: Pertaining to or characterized by hemorrhage.

hepatitis: Inflammation of the liver caused by bacterial invasion, chemical or physical agents, or viral infections; generally character- ized by an enlarged liver, fever, and jaundice accompanied by ab- normalities of liver function.

hepatitis B: A viral disease caused by the hepatitis B virus. It is endemic worldwide, and transmitted primarily by parenteral routes (e.g., blood transfusions, sharing of needles), intimate personal con- tact (e.g., sexual contact), and perinatally from mother to fetus. In the initial stage, there may be anorexia, fever, malaise, nausea, and vomiting. These decline with the onset of clinical jaundice, arthritis, and angioedema. Most patients recover completely.

hepatitis B virus (HBV): An unclassified DNA virus having com- plex, double-layered virions, a double-stranded genome, and three major antigens (the hepatitis B core antigen, surface antigen, and e antigen). It is the causative agent of hepatitis B.

hepatobiliary symptoms: Any perceptive change in the liver, bile, or biliary ducts indicating disease.

hepatomegaly: Enlargement of the liver.

herbal medicine: The science or art in which plants are used to prevent or cure disease and alleviate pain. Herbal medicine is based on a holistic approach to the patient, and relies on natural ingredi- ents including whole plants or parts of plants. The plants used typically have soft stems and contain little wood. The plants usually produce seeds, and then die down at the end of the growing season. *Also called* HERBALISM and PHYTOTHERAPY.

herbalism: *See* HERBAL MEDICINE.

heroin: *See* DIACETYLMORPHINE.

herpes encephalitis: Encephalitis due to infection with herpesvirus.

herpes simplex: An acute infectious disease caused by herpes sim- plex virus type 1 or 2. It is characterized by the development of one or more small, fluid-filled, thin-walled vesicles occurring as a primary infection or recurring because of reactivation of a latent infection. Type 1 infections generally do not involve genital areas of the body, whereas type 2 infections do. Acyclovir applied locally has been an effective form of treatment, with antibiotics often used to treat secondary infections.

herpes zoster: An acute infectious disease caused by the varicella-zoster virus. It is characterized by inflammation of the sensory ganglia. Severe neuralgic pain and vesicular eruption occur along the affected nerve. It is generally unilateral and is self-limited. It is believed that herpes zoster represents reactivation of latent varicella-zoster virus in individuals who previously presented with chicken pox and were rendered partially immune. *Also called* SHINGLES.

herpesvirus: Any one of a large group of DNA viruses important in humans, and found in many animal species. The viruses mature in the nucleus of the infected cell, where they cause the formation of a characteristic inclusion body (some cause the formation of a cytoplasmic inclusion body as well). Included in this group are herpes simplex virus type 1, herpes simplex virus type 2, cytomegalovirus, and Epstein-Barr virus.

heterosexual: (1) An individual whose sexual orientation is to persons of the opposite sex. (2) Pertaining to the opposite sex. (3) The opposite of HOMOSEXUAL. *Also called* STRAIGHT.

heterosexuality: Sexual attraction toward a person of the opposite sex.

high: (1) Intoxicated. (2) Under the influence of a drug or alcohol.

highly active antiretroviral therapy (HAART): Powerful combination of drugs, at least one of which is usually an HIV protease inhibitor. The goal of the therapy is to render HIV undetectable in the body of an infected person.

high-risk behavior: Any lifestyle choice or action that places an individual's health or well-being at increased risk. Where HIV is concerned, this most often involves unprotected sexual intercourse.

histidine: An amino acid obtained from tissue proteins. Histidine is necessary for tissue repair and growth.

histology: Study of the microscopic structure of tissue.

histopathology: The study of the microscopic structure of diseased tissues.

Histoplasma capsulatum: The causative agent of histoplasmosis which grows as a fungus and as a yeast. It occurs as small, oval, yeast-like cells in tissue, which appear to be encapsulated, but are not.

histoplasmosis: A respiratory disease due to the inhalation of *Histoplasma capsulatum*. Infection is generally asymptomatic. When symptoms appear, they range from a mild self-limited infection to severe illness (anemia, fever, acute pneumonia, leukopenia, enlargement of the spleen and liver, and gastrointestinal ulcers). It may be treated by administering amphotericin B intravenously.

history taking: (1) Systematically recording past events as they relate to a person or group of people. (2) Noting specific medical events that have occurred in a person's life, usually as part of a medical record.

HIV: *See* HUMAN IMMUNODEFICIENCY VIRUS.

HIV encephalitis: *See* AIDS DEMENTIA COMPLEX.

HIV encephalopathy: *See* AIDS DEMENTIA COMPLEX.

HIV wasting syndrome: The loss of weight and strength often accompanying infection with the human immunodeficiency virus that results in emaciation and enfeeblement. *Also called* SLIM DISEASE and WASTING SYNDROME.

HIV/AIDS Bureau of HRSA: Located within the Health Resources and Services Administration, the HIV/AIDS Bureau administers the Ryan White CARE Program and funds. HIV/AIDS Bureau of HRSA, Office of Communications, 5600 Fishers Lane, Room 7-46, Rockville MD 20857. Telephone: (301) 443-6652; Fax: (301) 443-0791; Web site, <http://www.hrsa.dhhs.gov/hab/default.htm>.

HIVID: *See* ZALCITABINE.

HIV-1: *See* HUMAN IMMUNODEFICIENCY VIRUS TYPE 1.

HIV-2: *See* HUMAN IMMUNODEFICIENCY VIRUS TYPE 2.

HL: *See* HAIRY LEUKOPLAKIA.

HLA: *See* HUMAN LEUKOCYTE ANTIGEN.

HMO: *See* HEALTH MAINTENANCE ORGANIZATION.

Hodgkin's disease: A form of malignant lymphoma of unknown cause that is characterized by painless, progressive enlargement of the lymph nodes, lymphoid tissue, liver, and spleen. Other symptoms may include anemia, anorexia, fever, night sweats, severe itching, and weight loss. It may appear as acute, localized, latent with relapsing fever, lymphogranulomatosis, and splenomegaly.

holistic health: The philosophy that an individual functions as a complete unit and cannot be reduced to the sum of his or her parts. Health then involves the whole person, not any particular organ system.

home care: The provision of health care in a patient's home. *Also called* HOME HEALTH CARE.

home health care: *See* HOME CARE.

home-based services: Any of a group of medical or social services delivered to, or administered at, an individual's home.

homeopathy: A system of medical practice that treats a disease with minute doses of a remedy that would produce symptoms of the disease in a healthy person.

homophobia: Fear of homosexuals or homosexuality.

homosexual: (1) An individual whose sexual orientation is toward persons of the same sex. (2) Pertaining to the same sex. (3) The opposite of heterosexual. *Also called* GAY.

homosexual sexual intercourse: Sexual union between individuals of the same sex.

homosexuality: Sexual attraction toward a person of the same sex.

hooker: *See* PROSTITUTE.

hospice: (1) An interdisciplinary approach to providing palliative and supportive care (economic, physical, social, and spiritual services) for the terminally ill. These services may be administered in a patient's home or a hospice facility. (2) A facility that provides palliative and supportive services for the terminally ill.

host: The organism (plant or animal) that harbors or nourishes a parasite.

hotline: Telephone assistance for providing crisis intervention to individuals experiencing severe problems (alcoholism, child abuse, spousal abuse, suicide, or rape). It is usually staffed continuously by paraprofessionals or professionals in the medical or social sciences. In the HIV/AIDS arena, hotlines also typically provide answers to questions about the disease, and serve as referral services to local service providers.

Housing and Civil Enforcement Section: A section of the Civil Rights Division, Department of Justice, the Housing and Civil Enforcement Section has responsibility for enforcing federal civil rights laws as they apply to the prohibition of discrimination in all housing transactions. Housing and Civil Enforcement Section, Civil Rights Division, Department of Justice, P.O. Box 65998, Washington, DC 20035. Telephone: (202) 514-4713; Fax: (202) 514-1116; Web site, <http://www.usdoj.gov/crt/crt-home.html>.

HPA-23: *See* ANTIMONIOTUNGSTATE.

HPMPC: *See* CIDOFOVIR.

HPV: *See* HUMAN PAPILLOMAVIRUS.

HRSA: *See* HEALTH RESOURCES AND SERVICES ADMINISTRATION.

HTLV: *See* HUMAN T-CELL LYMPHOTROPHIC VIRUS.

HTLV-III: *See* HUMAN T-CELL LEUKEMIA VIRUS III.

HUD: *See* DEPARTMENT OF HOUSING AND URBAN DEVELOPMENT.

human immunodeficiency virus (HIV): A retrovirus which infects the T4 lymphocyte cells, monocyte-macrophage cells, certain cell populations in the brain and spinal cord, and colorectal epithelial cells. HIV-infected cells weaken the immune system. However, individuals infected with the human immunodeficiency virus do not necessarily have AIDS. *Previously called* LYMPHADENOPATHY VIRUS, HUMAN T-CELL LEUKEMIA VIRUS III, and HUMAN T-CELL LYMPHOTROPHIC VIRUS III. *See also* ACQUIRED IMMUNODEFICIENCY SYNDROME.

human immunodeficiency virus type 1 (HIV-1): One of two main classes of the human immunodeficiency virus, considered to be more virulent than type 2. In the United States, HIV-1 is the most common form.

human immunodeficiency virus type 2 (HIV-2): One of two main classes of the human immunodeficiency virus, considered to be less virulent than type 1. Discovered in West Africa, it does not appear to be as prevalent in the United States as HIV-1.

human leukocyte antigen (HLA): The histocompatibility antigen governed by genes of the major human complex that controls the ability of cells to survive without immunological interference.

human papillomavirus (HPV): A subgroup of the papovaviruses causing papillomas or warts. *See also* ANAL WART and PAPOVAVIRUS.

human rights: That which belongs to a person by nature, tradition, law, or privilege.

human sexuality education: Education that increases the knowledge of the functional, structural, and behavioral aspects of human reproduction and sexual relationships.

human T-cell leukemia virus: *See* HUMAN T-CELL LYMPHOTROPHIC VIRUS.

human T-cell leukemia virus III (HTLV-III): *See* HUMAN IMMUNODEFICIENCY VIRUS.

human T-cell lymphotrophic virus (HTLV): A family of retroviruses that are lymphocytotrophic and particularly partial to T lymphocytes of the inducer/helper subset. *Also called* HUMAN T-CELL LEUKEMIA VIRUS.

humor therapy: Use of laughter to promote healing.

humoral abnormality: A deformity or deviation from the norm in body fluids (the antibody limb of protection).

humoral immunity: Immunity that is accomplished with the aid of antibodies.

hydrocodone: A narcotic analgesic drug related to codeine, but it is more potent and more addicting. The trade name is Vicodin.

hydrocortisone: The corticosteroid hormone produced by either the human adrenal cortex or synthetically. It is essential in maintaining life, sustaining blood pressure, and providing mineralocorticoid activity. Used in the treatment of various ailments (allergies, collagen abnormalities, inflammations, and certain neoplasms).

hydrogen peroxide: A colorless, syrupy liquid with an irritating odor and acrid taste. It may be used as a mild antiseptic, germicide, and cleansing agent as well as a commercial bleaching agent.

hydromorphone: An opioid analgesic drug made from morphine. The trade name is Dilaudid.

hydroxyzine: An antihistamine drug. Trade names are Atarax and Vistaril Parenteral.

hypercapnia: An excess of carbon dioxide in the blood.

hyperglycemia: An increased amount of sugar in the blood, resulting in a condition that may lower resistance to infection and may precede diabetic coma.

hypericin: A member of the plant family *Clusiaceae (Hypericaceae)*. Herbal and homeopathic preparations are used for depression, neuralgias, and a variety of other conditions. There is evidence that administration of hypericin in conjunction with indinavir significantly decreases the presence of the protease inhibitor in the bloodstream, causing indinavir to be considerably less effective and possibly promoting the development of viral resistance to the drug. Since other HIV/AIDS drugs are metabolized similarly to indinavir, patients using hypericin along with other medications are strongly urged to consult their primary care provider. *Also called* ST. JOHN'S WORT.

hyperkalemia: An increased amount of potassium in the blood, generally caused by defective renal excretion.

hyperplasia: An unusal increase in the number of normal cells in the normal tissue arrangement.

hypertension: A condition in which the patient has persistently high arterial blood pressure. The cause of hypertension may be unknown, or associated with the presence of other diseases.

hyperthermia: (1) Unusually high body temperature. (2) Therapy in which the body temperature is raised to an abnormal height to treat disease.

hypertrophy: The enlargement or growth of an organ or structure (not involving tumor formation) due to an increase in size of its constituent cells.

hypnosis: An induced state that resembles sleep, and in which the subject is responsive to the suggestions of the inducer.

hypnotherapy: Treatment by hypnosis or by inducing prolonged sleep.

hypodermic: Administered or inserted under the skin. It is used when a drug cannot be administered orally, readily absorbed in the gastrointestinal tract, or when gastrointestinal secretions would alter the drug. It may also be used to provide local anesthesia to the site of an injection.

hypoglycemia: A decreased amount of sugar in the blood. This condition may result in shakiness, cold sweat, fatigue, hypothermia, headache, and malaise. It may be accompanied by confusion, irritability, and weakness. Hypoglycemia may ultimately result in seizures, coma, and possibly death.

hypogonadism: A condition involving decreased functional activity and secretion of the gonads, resulting in slowed growth and sexual development or, in the adult, impairment of normal sexual function.

hypokalemia: A decreased amount of potassium in the circulating blood. It may result from a loss of potassium through renal secretion or through expulsion via the gastrointestinal tract (e.g., diarrhea or vomiting). Hypokalemia may be manifested by muscular weakness and paralysis, postural hypotension, renal disease, and gastrointestinal dysfunction.

hyponatremia: A decreased amount of sodium in the blood.

hypopharynx: The lowermost division of the pharynx, which lies below the epiglottis, and leads to the larynx and esophagus.

hypotension: A decrease in blood pressure below normal. It may be caused by dehydration, shock, fever, anemia, cancer, and various diseases. This may result in debilitation or wasting, and impending death.

hypothermia: Having a body temperature that is below normal. This may be due to prolonged exposure to extreme cold or may be induced artificially. Hypothermia is induced to lower the rate of metabolism thereby reducing oxygen need. Used in various surgical procedures, especially cardiovascular and neurological procedures.

hypovolemia: A decreased volume of blood in the body.

hypoxemia: Deficient oxygenation of the blood. *See also* HYPOXIA.

hypoxia: (1) A decreased amount of oxygen. (2) A decreased concentration of oxygen in the blood distributed to tissue.

hyssop: A European mint used in medicine. This herb is believed to regulate blood pressure, purify the blood, and promote circulation. It is also claimed to be an excellent aid for the eyes, hoarseness, lungs, mucous buildup, nervous disorders, and skin problems.

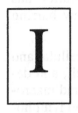

IAPAC: *See* INTERNATIONAL ASSOCIATION OF PHYSICIANS IN AIDS CARE.

ibuprofen: (1) An anti-inflammatory. (2) A nonsteroidal anti-inflammatory agent used in the treatment of osteoarthritis and rheumatoid arthritis. The trade names are Advil, Motrin, and Nuprin.

ichthyosis: A noninflammatory condition in which the skin is dry and scaly. Depending on the stage and degree of the condition, it has been described in terms of various animals (e.g., alligator skin, crocodile skin, fish skin).

ICL: *See* IDIOPATHIC CD4+T LYMPHOCYTOPENIA.

icterus: *See* JAUNDICE.

ICU: *See* INTENSIVE CARE UNIT.

idiopathic CD4+T lymphocytopenia (ICL): An immunodeficiency syndrome of unknown origin. ICL is sometimes referred to as non-HIV AIDS. As in AIDS patients, ICL patients exhibit reduced numbers of CD4+T lymphocytes. ICL patients may present with opportunistic infections as well, but ICL differs from HIV in its progression, because the CD4 T-cell counts remain stable.

idiopathic inflammatory pulmonary disease: A pathologic condition—causing inflammation of the lungs—of unknown origin, and not a result of any other disease.

idiopathic thrombocytopenic purpura (ITP): A form of a purpura, often accompanied by the presence of a serum antiplatelet antibody, unassociated with any definable systemic disease in which the blood platelet count is decreased.

IHS: *See* INDIAN HEALTH SERVICE.

IL-1: *See* INTERLEUKIN-1.

IL-2: *See* INTERLEUKIN-2.

imipramine: An antidepressant drug of the tricyclic class. The trade name is Tofranil.

immigration: Influx of individuals into one country from another one. In the context of the HIV/AIDS epidemic, immigration has been controversial since the U.S. Congress passed a law barring entry to all HIV-positive individuals.

immune system: A complex system made up of various cellular and molecular components that distinguishes self from not self, and defends the body against foreign substances. Lymphocytes and macrophages are the primary cellular components; antibodies and lymphokines constitue the primary molecular components. Granulocytes and the complement system are involved in immune responses, but they are not necessarily considered part of the immune system.

immune system abnormality: A deviation in the normal functioning of the immune system.

immune thrombocytopenic purpura: A form of purpura occurring as a consequence of a disturbance in the immune system (e.g., infection with the human immunodeficiency virus) in which the platelet count is decreased.

immunity: (1) The state or condition of being protected from a disease, especially an infectious one. It is usually induced by immunization, previous infection, or by other nonimmunologic factors. (2) The response of the body and its tissues to a variety of antigens including pollens, red cells, transplanted tissues, or the individual's own cells.

immunization: Becoming immune; inducing immunity; rendering a patient immune.

immunodeficiency: A compromised or decreased ability to respond to antigenic stimuli. It is classified as antibody, cellular, combined deficiency, or phagocytic dysfunction disorders. *See also* ACQUIRED IMMUNODEFICIENCY SYNDROME.

immunoflourescence assay: The detection of antibodies by using special proteins labeled with fluorescein. If the specific organism or antibody that is being searched for is present, it is observed as a fluorescent material when examined microscopically while illuminated with a fluorescent light source.

immunology: The branch of science dealing with the study of immunity.

immunopathogenesis: A process in which the course of a disease is affected/altered by an immune response or by the products of an immune response.

immunosuppression: The prevention or diminution of the formation of immune response.

impetigo: A contagious, inflammatory skin disease caused by direct inoculation of Group A streptococci or *Staphylococcus aureus* into superficial cutaneous abrasions or compromised skin. It is marked by isolated pustules that rupture to discharge an amber-colored fluid composed of serum and pus; the fluid dries to form a thick, yellowish crust. The pustules may spread peripherally, but they are usually found around the nose and mouth.

impotence: (1) The inability of the male to achieve or maintain penile erection. (2) Weakness.

Imreg: A natural leukocyte-derived, polypeptide immunomodulator that has been shown to enhance production of certain lymphokines in the laboratory.

Imuran: *See* AZATHIOPRINE.

imuthiol: An organic compound that contains sulfur, and is an inducer of T lymphocytes. It has been shown to have anti-HIV activity in vitro.

in vitro: Within a glass; in an artificial environment.

in vitro cultivation: The propagation of living organisms in an artificial environment such as a petri dish or test tube.

in vivo: Within the living body; in a living organism.

inactivation agent: An agent used to destroy biological activity, as of an enzyme, microorganism, or virus (e.g., heat).

INAPEN: *See* INTERNATIONAL AIDS PROSPECTIVE EPIDEMIOLOGY NETWORK.

Inapsine: *See* DROPERIDOL.

incidence: (1) The rate of new occurrence of any event over a period of time in relation to the population within which it occurs (i.e, the number of new cases of a disease). (2) The act or manner of falling upon or influencing.

incontinence: (1)The inability to control excretory functions (e.g., feces, semen, urine). (2) The absence of restraint; immoderation or excess.

incubation: (1) The interval between exposure to a pathogen and the appearance of the first clinical symptom in the development of an infectious disease. (2) The development of bacterial culture under controlled conditions. (3) The development of a fertilized egg. (4) The care of a premature infant in a controlled environment (humidity, oxygen, temperature) to promote development and survival.

incubation period: The latent interval during which an infection or disease is present without manifesting itself.

IND: *See* INVESTIGATIONAL NEW DRUG.

indeterminate test: Results of a test for HIV antibodies wherein it is impossible to determine whether the individual is negative or positive. Tests should be repeated as soon as possible to determine status.

index case: The initial individual whose state of health prompted investigation into a disorder.

Index Medicus: See CUMULATED INDEX MEDICUS.

Indian Health Service (IHS): The IHS is the agency primarily responsible, at the federal level, for the health care and health advocacy for all Native American and Alaskan native populations in the

United States. Health services designed to be culturally appropriate are provided to more than 1.5 million people in 34 states. Listed on the Web site, <http://www.ihs.gov.>, is complete contact information for all twelve regional offices of the Indian Health Service. To contact the Washington, DC area office, write or call the Communications Staff, Indian Health Service, Room 6-35, Parklawn Building, 5600 Fishers Road, Rockville MD 20857. Telephone: (301) 443-3593; Fax: (301) 443-0507.

indinavir: A potent and specific HIV protease inhibitor that appears to have good oral bioavailability. The trade name is Crixivan.

individual masturbation: Gratification of sexual desires when one is alone. *See also* MUTUAL MASTURBATION.

individual psychological treatment models: Any of a group of psychological treatment modalities, administered on an individual basis, designed to foster mental health and well-being.

Individual Treatment IND: A program established by the Food and Drug Administration (FDA) in which a person may receive an experimental drug free of charge from the pharmaceutical manufacturer with the assistance of a personal physician. Admission to this program is granted on an individual basis by the FDA. *See also* INVESTIGATIONAL NEW DRUG.

induced hyperthermia: Fever artificially produced to favorably modify the course of a disease.

induced immunosuppression: The prevention or diminution of an immune response by artificial means.

indurate: (1) To harden. (2) Hardened.

infant: A liveborn child from birth through one year of age. *See also* NEONATE.

infection: The state or condition in which the body or part of it is invaded by microorganisms. The microorganisms will multiply under favorable conditions, producing injurious results. If the body's defense mechanisms are effective, the infection will remain localized. If the body's defense mechanisms are not capable of staving off the invasion and multiplication, the local infection may persist and spread.

infectious agent: (1) Something that produces infection. (2) Something that is capable of being transmitted with or without contact.

infectious mononucleosis: An acute infectious disease that primarily affects lymphoid tissue, and is characterized by enlarged lymph nodes and spleen with an increase in abnormal mononuclear leukocytes in the blood. It is associated with Epstein-Barr virus.

inflammatory bowel disease: A general term used to denote those inflammatory diseases of the bowel of unknown origin (e.g., ulcerative colitis, Chrohn's disease, regional enteritis).

inflammatory neuropathy: Inflammation of the peripheral nervous system causing abnormal function.

influenza: An acute, contagious, respiratory infection characterized by sudden onset, fever, chills, headache, muscle pain, and sometimes exhaustion. Cough and sore throat are common. It is usually self-limiting and lasts 2 to 7 days.

influenza virus vaccine: A sterile suspension of killed influenza virus types A and B, either individually or combined. Annual immunization before November is recommended for high-risk individuals. Trade names are Fluax and Fluogen.

informed consent: Permission that is voluntarily granted for any medical procedure, test, or medication by a competent individual. It is based on an understanding of the alternatives, nature, risks, and possible benefits involved.

injection drug use: Drug abuse by injecting intramuscularly or under the skin.

inositol: A sugar-like crystalline substance found in the liver, kidney, skeletal, and heart muscle; it is also present in the leaves and seeds of most plants. It is part of the vitamin B complex.

inpatient services: Any of a group of medical or social support services provided to individuals while hospitalized.

insertive anal intercourse: Sexual intercourse in which the individual inserts the penis into the anus of his partner. *Also called* ACTIVE ANAL INTERCOURSE.

insomnia: Prolonged or abnormal sleeplessness.

insulin: A protein hormone secreted by beta cells of the pancreas. Insulin plays a major role in the regulation of glucose metabolism, generally promoting the cellular utilization of glucose. It is also an important regulator of protein and lipid metabolism. Insulin is used as a drug to control insulin-dependent diabetes mellitus.

insurance: (1) The business of insuring persons or property. (2) Coverage by contract whereby one party agrees to indemnify or guarantee another against loss by a specified contingent event or peril.

intensive care: Service provided by skilled medical personnel to seriously ill patients requiring special equipment and continuous attention. It is usually provided in a designated area of the care facility (e.g., intensive care unit).

intensive care unit (ICU): A designated area within the care facility that provides special equipment and continuous attention by medical personnel to the seriously ill.

intercourse: Interaction between individuals or groups. *See also* SEXUAL INTERCOURSE, HOMOSEXUAL SEXUAL INTERCOURSE, ANAL INTERCOURSE, INSERTIVE ANAL INTERCOURSE, RECEPTIVE ANAL INTERCOURSE, and VAGINAL INTERCOURSE.

interferon: Any of the glycoproteins formed when cells are exposed to viral or other foreign nucleic acids and which exert host-specific but not viral-specific antiviral activities. Interferons are important in immune function, have antitumor activity, and can repress the growth of nonviral parasites within the cells.

interleukin-1 (IL-1): A substance produced by macrophages that induces the production of interleukin-2 by T cells that have been stimulated by antigen or mitogen.

interleukin-2 (IL-2): A lymphokine produced by T cells in response to antigenic or mitogenic stimulation and the signal carried by interleukin-1. It stimulates the growth and proliferation of T lymphocytes, and is used as an anticancer drug. The side effects are sometimes fatal.

interment: Burial.

internal medicine: *See* GENERAL INTERNAL MEDICINE.

Internal Revenue Service (IRS): Housed within the Department of the Treasury, the IRS offers special help and problem resolution lines for people with disabilities. Problem Resolution Hotline: (877) 777-4778, TDD: (800) 829-4059 (English/Spanish); Web site, <http://www.irs.ustreas.gov/>.

International AIDS Prospective Epidemiology Network (INAPEN): Founded in 1984, this organization seeks to heighten the effectiveness of research in the AIDS arena by promoting cooperation, data sharing, and standardization of research methodologies. In addition to fostering collaborative research, it maintains biographical archives and compiles statistics to aid in research. International AIDS Prospective Epidemiology Network, 155 N. Harbor Drive, No. 5103, Chicago, IL 60601. Telephone: (312) 565-2109.

International Association of Physicians in AIDS Care (IAPAC): Founded in 1995, IAPAC provides educational programs to care-givers, physicians, and patients. The Association publishes the *Journal of the International Association of Physicians in AIDS Care.* International Association of Physicians in AIDS Care, 225 West Washington Street, Suite 2200, Chicago, IL 60606. Telephone: (312) 419-7295; e-mail: iapac@aol.com. Web site, <http://www.iapac.org>.

Internet: A group of computer communication networks around the world. The networks that make up the Internet are connected through several backbone networks. The Internet was designed to facilitate information exchange.

intertriginous infection: (1) Inflammation occurring in the folds of the skin. (2) A superficial dermatitis occurring in the folds of the skin such as the creases in the neck, between the toes, or the groin. It is characterized by redness, maceration, burning, itching, and occasionally ulceration and erosion.

intertrigo: A form of dematitis occurring on skin surfaces that are in contact with each other, such as the creases or folds on the neck, or between the toes. The condition is caused by moisture and friction.

intertrigo labialis: *See* PERLECHE.

intestinal malabsorption: *See* CELIAC DISEASE.

intracranial disorders: Any pathological condition situated within the skull.

intrahepatic disease: Any pathological condition within the liver, which produces a group of clinical symptoms peculiar to it and that sets it apart as abnormal.

intrapartum: Occurring during childbirth or delivery.

intrathecal: (1) Within the spinal cord. (2) Within a sheath.

intrathoracic adenopathy: Swelling of the gland or lymph nodes within the chest.

intravenous (IV): Within, or into, a vein or veins.

intravenous drug abuser (IVDA): *See* INTRAVENOUS DRUG USER.

intravenous drug user (IVDU): An individual who uses, or over-uses, any drug that is injected into a vein in a manner that deviates from the drug's intended use. *Also called* INTRAVENOUS DRUG ABUS-ER (IVDA).

intubation: The insertion of a tube into a body canal or any hollow organ (e.g., the trachea to permit the entrance of air).

invasive nutritional substitute: Any nutrient administered intrave-nously.

invasive procedure: A technique involving the puncture of the skin or the insertion of foreign matter by using a device, needle, or tube to enter the body.

Investigational New Drug (IND): The status provided by the Food and Drug Administration that allows a compound to be tested on humans for the first time. *See also* INDIVIDUAL TREATMENT IND.

Invirase: *See* SAQUINAVIR.

iodine: A nonmetallic halogen essential in nutrition. It is especially necessary for the synthesis of thyroid hormones, which regulate the metabolic rate of cells. It is used in solution as a topical anti-infec-tive agent.

iodoquinol: An antiamebic agent appearing as a yellowish to tan crystalline powder. It is used in the treatment of amebiasis and

Trichomonas hominis infection of the intestine, and *Trichomonas vaginalis* vaginitis. It is administered orally in the treatment of intestinal disorders and intravaginally for vaginitis. The trade name is *Yodoxin*. *Also called* DIIODOHYDROXYQUIN.

IPV: *See* POLIOVIRUS VACCINE INACTIVATED.

iron: A metallic element found in certain minerals, nearly all soils, and mineral waters. Iron is an essential component of hemaglobin, cytochrome, and other components of respiratory enzyme systems. Iron transports oxygen to tissues and aids in cellular oxidation.

IRS: *See* INTERNAL REVENUE SERVICE.

ischemia: Local deficiency of blood supply due to functional constriction or actual obstruction of a blood vessel.

ischemic: Pertaining to, or affected with, ischemia.

isoleucine: An essential amino acid found in small amounts in most proteins.

isoniazid: An odorless, antibacterial compound appearing as colorless or white crystals, or as a white crystalline powder. Isoniazid is used in the treatment of tuberculosis. It may be administered orally or intramuscularly. The trade names are Dinacrin and Nydrazid.

Isoprinosine: An immunomodulator that enhances certain cell-mediated immune functions. It has been shown to have anti-HIV activity in vitro. The drug is available without prescription in several countries including Mexico. Although it has been popular for self-treatment, isoprinosine's antiviral effects have not consistently correlated with clinical improvement.

Isospora belli **infection:** Invasion of the body by a species of coccidian protozoa that parasitize the small intestine. Infection is known as coccidiosis. It is generally asymptomatic. When symptoms appear, they may manifest in severe, watery mucous diarrhea. *See also* COCCIDIOSIS.

itch: (1) Irritation of the skin, inducing the desire to scratch. (2) Marked by pruritus. (3) Any of a variety of skin disorders characterized by itching. (4) Scabies.

ITP: *See* IMMUNE THROMBOCYTOPENIC PURPURA.

itraconazole: An antifungal agent that has been used in the treatment of histoplasmosis, blastomycosis, cryptococcal meningitis, and aspergillosis. The trade name is Sporanox.

IV: *See* INTRAVENOUS.

IVDA: *See* INTRAVENOUS DRUG USER.

IVDU: *See* INTRAVENOUS DRUG USER.

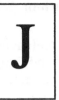

jaundice: A condition characterized by the yellow appearance of the skin, mucous membranes, whites of the eyes, and body fluids. It is caused by the deposition of bile pigment resulting from too much bilirubin in the blood. *Also called* ICTERUS.

john: (1) A customer of a prostitute. (2) Any easy mark.

Joint United Nations Program on AIDS (UNAIDS): This program is the 1996 successor to the Global Programme on AIDS. In an effort to advocate more effectively, use UN system resources more economically, and lend greater coherence to UN support of AIDS programs in countries throughout the world, six United Nations agencies joined forces to combat the pandemic. The agencies include the United Nations Children's Fund (UNICEF), the United Nations Development Program (UNDP), the United Nations Population Fund (UNFPA), the United Nations Educational, Scientific and Cultural Organization (UNESCO), the World Health Organization (WHO), and the World Bank.

kambucha tea: *See* KOMBUCHA TEA.

Kampo medicine: System of herbal medicine practiced in Japan by both herbalists and practitioners of modern medicine. Kampo originated in China and is based on Chinese herbal medicine. *See also* ORIENTAL TRADITIONAL MEDICINE and CHINESE TRADITIONAL MEDICINE.

Kaposi's sarcoma (KS): Neoplasms, which generally manifest with lymph node involvement or mucocutaneous lesions, particularly in the oral cavity or on the face. Lesions are usually red or purple, may assume varied shapes (round or elliptical), and do not pale under pressure. Internal lesions, especially in the gastrointestinal tract, occur in approximately half of those infected but are most often clinically silent. Neoplasms are generally painless at the outset but may become painful as lesions become more extensive. Therapy is controversial.

Kaposi's Sarcoma Research and Education Foundation: *See* SAN FRANCISCO AIDS FOUNDATION.

Kefauver amendments: Named after Senator Estes Kefauver, these amendments were passed in 1962 to force the Food and Drug Administration to ensure that drugs were both effective and safe.

ketoconazole: A broad-spectrum, antifungal agent administered orally, and used in the treatment of a variety of cutaneous fungal infections. The brand name is Nizoral.

kinesiology: The science or study of human muscular movement, especially in physical education and exercise physiology.

kiss: (1) A touch or caress with the lips given as an expression of affection, desire, or greeting. It may be with or without pressure and suction. (2) To touch or caress with the lips as an expression of affection, desire, or greeting. *See also* FRENCH KISS.

kitchen sink therapy: Use of all drugs possible by patients whose illnesses have not responded to standard regimens. *See also* SALVAGE THERAPY.

Klonopin: *See* CLONAZEPAM.

kombucha tea: A beverage derived from kombucha, a culture consisting of various yeasts and bacteria, and fermented with sweetened tea. It is believed to contain health-enhancing vitamins, enzymes, minerals, and organic acids.

KS: *See* KAPOSI'S SARCOMA.

Kuru disease: A rare disease of the central nervous system isolated in natives of the eastern New Guinea highlands. It is characterized at the onset by a disturbance in muscle coordination that progresses to paralysis, dementia, and eventual death. The incidence rate of Kuru has steadily declined in eastern New Guinea natives since the end (c. 1960) of the ritualistic practice of cannibalism (including the brain of the deceased). *See also* CREUTZFELDT-JAKOB DISEASE.

Kytril: *See* GRANISETRON.

L

Lactobacillus casei **factor:** *See* FOLIC ACID.

Lambda Legal Defense and Education Fund: This fund was founded in 1973 to protect the rights of homosexuals in areas such as the acquired immunodeficiency syndrome, the administration of justice, child custody, education, employment, and housing; it seeks to achieve its goal by engaging in test case litigation, presenting statistics and theoretical information to the court, educating the court as to the needs of homosexuals, educating the gay community about legal rights, and providing assistance to attorneys. The fund maintains a national network of participating attorneys, operates a speakers' bureau, and sponsors various seminars. Lambda Legal Defense and Education Fund, 120 Wall Street, Suite 1500, New York, NY 10005. Telephone: (212) 809-8585.

Lamblia intestinalis: *See* GIARDIA LAMBLIA.

lambliasis: *See* GIARDIASIS.

lamivudine (3TC): A reverse transcriptase inhibitor used to treat HIV disease. The trade name is Epivir.

Langerhans cell: A star-shaped dendritic cell found primarily in the epidermis. Langerhans cells are believed to be antigen-presenting cells, thus participating in certain immune responses.

LAS: *See* LYMPHADENOPATHY SYNDROME.

Lasagna Committee hearings: *See* NATIONAL COMMITTEE TO REVIEW CURRENT PROCEDURES FOR APPROVAL OF NEW DRUGS FOR CANCER AND AIDS.

laser surgery: The use of a laser either to vaporize surface lesions or to make bloodless cuts in tissue.

laser therapy: Treatment, in surgical procedures, using a device that converts various frequencies of light into a single, small, intense, unified beam of monochromatic radiation.

Lassa fever: A disease caused by arenavirus. A native African rat species is a common carrier. Symptoms include acute high fever, abdominal and chest pain, headache, dizziness, coughing, nausea, diarrhea, and vomiting. The skin and mucous membranes may begin to hemorrhage. Lassa fever has a relatively high mortality rate in Africa.

latex agglutination test: A test using latex particles as passive carriers of absorbed antigens. The particles clump together after a specific antibody is added.

latex condom: Covering for the penis made of latex. Latex and polyurethane condoms offer protection against sexually transmitted diseases including HIV.

LAV: *See* LYMPHADENOPATHY ASSOCIATED VIRUS.

laying on of hands: *See* THERAPEUTIC TOUCH.

L-carnitine: A naturally occurring amino acid that nourishes and strengthens muscles, and nutritionally supports the circulatory system.

lecithin: Any of several phosphatides found in milk, egg yolks, soybeans, corn, etc. These phosphatides are also found in blood and nerve tissue. Lecithin is used as a wetting, emulsifying, or penetrating agent.

legal assistance services: Any of a group of support services designed to provide legal advice or assistance to those in need.

Legionella pneumophila: A species of gram-negative bacteria that causes Legionnaires' disease and Pontiac fever. It has been isolated from numerous locations including tap water, soil, cooling-tower water, aerosolized droplets from heat-exchange systems, human lung tissue, respiratory secretions, and blood.

lentivirus: Any of a group of retroviruses, including those that cause certain diseases in sheep, which affect the pulmonary and central nervous systems.

leprosy: A chronic infectious disease caused by *Mycobacterium leprae*. It progresses slowly and may manifest itself in various clinical forms. The two principal, or polar, forms are lepromatous and tuberculoid. The lepromatous form is characterized by the development of lesions in the skin and symmetrical involvement of the peripheral nerves, which yields skin anesthesia, muscle weakness, and paralysis. The lepromatous form tends to involve the skin, respiratory tract, and testes. In the tuberculoid form, skin anesthesia occurs early and the nerve lesions are asymmetrical. This form is usually benign. Lepromatous leprosy is much more contagious and malignant than tuberculoid leprosy. Between these two polar forms are the borderline and indeterminant types of leprosy. The borderline form possesses clinical and bacteriological features representing a combination of the two polar forms. The indeterminant group presents fewer skin lesions and less abundant bacteria in the lesions.

lesbian: (1) An individual who practices lesbianism. (2) A woman whose sexual orientation is toward other women. *Also called* DYKE. *See also* HOMOSEXUAL.

lesbianism: Homosexual practice between women. Lesbianism was named after the Island of Lesbos, where the practice of lesbianism was reputed to have been common. *Also called* sapphism after Sappho, the early Sixth century B.C. Greek lyric poet who lived on the Island of Lesbos.

lesion: (1) Any pathologically altered, circumscribed area of tissue. (2) An infected area of skin.

leucine: An essential amino acid produced by the hydrolysis of proteins by pancreatic enzymes during digestion, and by the putrefaction of nitrogenous organic matter.

leucovorin: *See* FOLINIC ACID.

leukemia: A chronic or acute disease of the blood-forming elements characterized by the unrestrained growth of leukocytes and their precursors in the blood and bone marrow. Leukemia is classified on the basis of the dominant cell type involved.

leukocyte: A white blood cell or corpuscle. Leukocytes may be classified into two main groups: granulocytes and agranulocytes (nongranular). Granulocytes possess granules in their cytoplasm; they include neutrophils, eosinophils, and basophils. Agranulocytes do not possess granules in their cytoplasm; they include monocytes and lymphocytes.

leukoencephalopathy: Any of a group of diseases affecting the white matter of the brain.

leukopenia: An abnormal reduction of white blood corpuscles (leukocytes), usually below 5,000 per cubic millimeter. Leukopenia may be caused by various infections, drugs, or bone marrow failure.

leukoplakia: A disease characterized by white patches that will not rub off. Typically involves mucous membranes such as the tongue or gums.

Levo-Dromoran: *See* LEVORPHANOL.

Levoprome: *See* METHOTRIMEPRAZINE.

levorphanol: A narcotic analgesic that may be habit-forming. It may be administered orally or subcutaneously.

liability: (1) The state of being legally bound or obligated. (2) The debts of a person or business.

licorice: The dried root of a European perennial plant of the pea family, with spikes of blue flowers and short, flat pods. May also refer to a black extract made from the root. It is used as a vehicle and diluting agent or as a flavoring.

life cycle: The series of changes in form undergone by any developing organism, from its earliest stage to the recurrence of that same stage in the subsequent generation.

Lioresal: *See* BACLOFEN.

lipids: Any of a group of organic compounds consisting of the fats and other substances of similar properties. They are important constituents of living cells.

liposome: A spherical particle in an aqueous medium, formed by a lipid bilayer enclosing an aqueous compartment.

Listeria monocytogenes: A species of gram-positive bacteria. In humans, it produces such disorders as meningitis and perinatal septicemia.

liver *Lactobacillus casei* factor: *See* FOLIC ACID.

living will: A document detailing a person's wishes regarding artificial life support in the event of impending death. This document is drawn up while the person is of sound mind. Living wills are not legal in all states. *See also* DURABLE POWER OF ATTORNEY, MEDICAL DIRECTIVE, and NO CODE.

long-term survivor: An HIV-positive person who has progressed to AIDS but who remains relatively free of opportunistic infections, and other complications commonly experienced by individuals with ravaged immune systems.

lorazepam: An antianxiety agent with few side effects. It also has hypnotic, anticonvulsant, and considerable sedative properties.

Lotrimin: *See* CLOTRIMAZOLE.

low-risk behavior: Behavior that poses little risk for transmission of HIV or other blood-borne pathogens. Frottage is an example of low-risk behavior.

lubricant: A substance used to coat the anal or vaginal canal to ease insertion of a partner's fingers, hands, penis, or sex toy.

Ludiomil: *See* MAPROTILINE.

lumbar puncture: A procedure performed for one of three reasons: to administer anesthetic, to measure cerebrospinal fluid pressure, or to withdraw a sample of cerebrospinal fluid for diagnostic purposes. The procedure consists of inserting an aspiration needle into the space of the spinal cord. Also called spinal puncture.

lumbosacral polyradiculopathy: Any of a group of diseases affecting the nerve roots in the lumbar vertebrae and the sacrum (low back region).

lupus anticoagulant: An acquired coagulation inhibitor first noted in patients with systemic lupus erythematosus, but it has since been found in association with other immune disorders, neoplastic disorders, myeloproliferative disorders, pregnancy, and secondary to the administration of certain drugs.

lymphadenopathy: Any disease process in which the lymph nodes are affected and abnormally enlarged.

lymphadenopathy associated virus (LAV): *See* HUMAN IMMUNO-DEFICIENCY VIRUS.

lymphadenopathy syndrome (LAS): A condition characterized by the presence of unexplained lymphadenopathy for 3 months or longer. Biopsy reveals nonspecific lymphoid hyperplasia. It is considered by some to be a prodrome (a warning symptom indicating the onset of disease) for the acquired immunodeficiency syndrome.

lymphoblast: A cell that gives rise to a lymphocyte.

lymphocyte: Any of the mononuclear, nonphagocytic leukocytes that make up the body's immunologically competent cells. Found in the blood, lymph, and lymphoid tissues, they are divided on the basis of function and ontogeny. The two main classes are B lymphocytes and T lymphocytes. B lymphocytes are responsible for humoral immunity; T lymphocytes are responsible for cellular immunity. Most are small, with an average of 10 to 12 micrometers in diameter.

lymphocytic interstitial pneumonitis: An inflammation within the lungs that develops gradually and is characterized by infiltration of the lungs by lymphocytes, lymphoblasts, and plasma cells. The cause is unknown, but it is often associated with a compromised immune system. *Also called* LYMPHOID INTERSTITIAL PNEUMONIA.

lymphoid interstitial pneumonia: *See* LYMPHOCYTIC INTERSTITIAL PNEUMONITIS.

lymphokine: A general term used to denote substances, released by sensitized lymphocytes on contact with antigen, that are soluble mediators of immune response. They stimulate macrophages and monocytes, assisting with cellular immunity.

lymphoma: A general term used to denote any neoplastic disorder in the lymphatic system. Diseases included under this general group are Hodgkin's disease, lymphatic leukemia, and reticuloses. The term lymphoma is frequently used to denote malignant lymphoma.

lymphoproliferative disease: *See* LYMPHOPROLIFERATIVE DISORDER.

lymphoproliferative disorder: Any of a group of malignant neoplasms which involve lymphoreticular cells. Included are such disorders as Hodgkin's disease, lymphocytic lymphomas, multiple myelomas, and the histiocytic, lymphocytic, and monocytic leukemias. *Also called* lymphoproliferative disease and lymphoproliferative syndrome.

lymphoproliferative syndrome: *See* LYMPHOPROLIFERATIVE DISORDER.

lymphoreticular cell: Any reticuloendothelial cell of the lymph node.

lymphotrophic: Having an affinity for lymphatic tissue.

lysine: An essential amino acid obtained synthetically or by the hydrolysis of certain proteins in digestion.

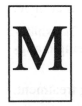

ma haung: A Chinese herb believed to be effective in treating asthma and in reducing upper respiratory infections. Primary active ingredient is ephedra.

macrobiotic diet: A special selection of food and drink designed with the intention of prolonging life. The standard macrobiotic diet recommends that food intake be as follows: 50 percent whole cereal grains, 20 to 30 percent vegetables, 5 to 10 percent soups, and 5 to 10 percent beans and sea vegetables. Elimination of all meat except occasional fish, animal fat, eggs, poultry, and dairy products is part of a macrobiotic regimen.

macrophage: Any of the various forms of mononuclear phagocytes found in loose connective tissues and many organs of the body. Functions of macrophages include nonspecific phagocytosis and pinocytosis, specific pinocytosis of microorganisms that facilitate phagocytosis, killing of ingested microorganisms, digestion and distribution of antigens to B and T lymphocytes, and secretion of various products (e.g., enzymes, prostaglandins, interferon, interleukin-1, complement components, and coagulation factors).

magnesium: A light, silvery, metallic element. Its salts are essential in nutrition as they are required for the activity of many enzymes, especially those concerned with oxidative breakdown of glycogen and other complex sugars.

magnetic resonance imaging (MRI): A technique for providing images of the soft tissues of the body (e.g., heart, brain, large blood vessels) by applying a strong, external, magnetic field that allows for distinguishing between hydrogen atoms in different environments. *Also called* NUCLEAR MAGNETIC RESONANCE IMAGING (NMRI).

MAI: *See* MYCOBACTERIUM AVIUM-INTRACELLULARE.

malabsorption syndromes: A general term for syndromes of malnutrition due to the failure of normal intestinal absorption of nutrients.

male-to-female transmission: (1) Sexual transmission of a communicable disease from a male to a female. (2) The passage or transfer of any pathologic condition from one male to a female.

male-to-male transmission: (1) Sexual transmission of a communicable disease from one male to another male. (2) The passage or transfer of any pathologic condition from one male to another male.

malignancy: (1) A tumor or neoplasm that is not benign. (2) Exhibiting a tendency to progress in virulence. (3) The state of being malignant.

malignant: (1) Becoming progressively worse; resisting treatment. (2) Tending to produce death; harmful.

malnutrition: (1) Any disorder of nutrition. (2) The deficit of efficient or substantive food substances in the body, or the inability to properly absorb food substances and distribute them throughout the body.

mammography: Use of radiography of the breast to diagnose cancer.

managed care: Health insurance intended to reduce unnecessary health care costs through a variety of mechanisms including economic incentives for physicians and patients to select less costly forms of care; programs for reviewing the necessity of specific medical services; increased beneficiary cost-sharing controls on inpatient admissions and length of stays; selective contracting with health care providers; cost sharing incentives for outpatient surgery; and the intensive management of high cost health care cases.

mandatory testing: Testing or screening required by federal, state, or local laws or other agencies for the diagnosis of specified conditions.

manganese: A metal element found in many foods, plants, and in the tissue of the higher animals. Manganese is an essential element needed for normal bone metabolism and many enzyme reactions. It is an antioxidant nutrient, and is important for the production of energy.

mange: (1) A skin disease in mammals characterized by itching, lesions, scabs, and loss of hair caused by parasitic mites. (2) A cutaneous communicable disease occurring in various animals including dogs, cats, cattle, horses, sheep, rabbits, rats, and some birds. The causative agent is any of several of the mange mites including *Chorioptes*, *Demodex*, *Psoroptes*, and *Sarcoptes*. In humans, this condition is known as scabies.

mange mite: Any of the various mites which cause mange.

manual intercourse: Gratification of sexual desire accomplished by the insertion of a hand into the vaginal canal or anus.

MAP: *See* MOTHERS OF AIDS PATIENTS.

maprotiline: An antidepressant drug. The trade name is Ludiomil.

Marburg: Virulent hemorrhagic virus first recognized in Marburg, Germany. Marburg is a filovirus.

marijuana: *See* CANNABIS.

Marinol: *See* DRONABINOL.

masochism: (1) Deriving sexual pleasure from being dominated, mistreated, or physically abused by one's partner. (2) Deriving pleasure from suffering physical or psychological pain. (3) The opposite of sadism.

massage: Therapeutic manipulation of the major muscle groups of the human body. Several different techniques for massage have been developed including Swedish and shiatsu.

mastitis: Inflammation or infection of the breast or mammary gland.

mastoiditis: Inflammation or infection of the air cells of the nipple-shaped portion of the temporal bone (mastoid process).

masturbation: Self-stimulation of the genitals, or other erogenous zones, for sexual pleasure. The term usually applies to self-stimulation to the point of orgasm.

Maternal AIDS Project: A project of the Health Care Financing Administration, the Maternal AIDS Project was developed to increase both patient and provider knowledge about drugs that reduce the transmission of HIV from mother to fetus, and about the availability of Medicaid coverage for prenatal care. Director, Division of Advocacy and Special Issues, HCFA—Center for Medicaid and State Operations, 7500 Security Boulevard, Baltimore MD 21244. Telephone: (410) 786-1357; Web site, <http://www.hcfa.gov/hiv/default.htm>.

Maternal and Child Health Bureau (MCHB): A bureau within the Health Resources and Services Administration (HRSA), the MCHB administers a discretionary grants program for local projects that seek to reduce infant mortality, and improve the health of children and families by developing public-private partnerships. The MCHB also provides national leadership to both public and private sectors concerned with the delivery of health care services to mothers and children. Maternal and Child Health Bureau, 5600 Fishers Lane, Parklawn Building, Room 13A-54, Rockville, MD 20857. Telephone: (301) 443-0767; Fax: (301) 443-4842; Web site, <http://www.mchb.hrsa.gov/>.

mechanical ventilation: The process of exchanging air between the lungs and surrounding atmosphere by artificial, extrinsic means (e.g., respirator).

Medicaid: The U.S. government program designed to provide medical services to the needy and medically needy. It operates through grants to states, and is overseen by the Health Care Financing Administration. Administrator, Health Care Financing Administration, Department of Health and Human Services, 200 Independence Avenue S.W., Washington, DC 20201. Telephone: (410) 786-3151.

medical assistance services: Support services designed to provide health care to those in need.

medical directive: A document detailing a patient's wishes concerning the kinds of treatment he or she does not wish to have administered. *See also* CODE-BLUE STATUS, DURABLE POWER OF ATTORNEY, LIVING WILL, NO CODE.

Medicare: The federal health insurance program administered by the Health Care Financing Administration. It is designed to provide medical and hospital care to the elderly (persons over 65), and certain disabled persons such as those with end-stage renal disease. Medicare is funded through social security contributions, premiums, and general revenue. Administrator, Health Care Financing Administration, Department of Health and Human Services, 200 Independence Avenue S.W., Washington, DC 20201. Telephone: (410) 786-3151.

medicinal plants: Any of a variety of plants, including herbs, that are used to relieve pain or cure disease.

meditation: (1) The act of reflection or contemplation. (2) Deep, continued thought. (3) Solemn reflection on matters as a devotional act. *See also* MYSTICISM.

Megace: *See* MEGESTROL ACETATE.

megaloblast: A large, abnormal, red blood corpuscle, which is oval and slightly irregular in shape, from 11 to 20 microns in diameter. It can be classified as basophilic, orthochromatic, or polychromatic.

megaloblastic anemia: Anemia characterized by the presence of megaloblasts in the blood and bone marrow.

megestrol acetate: A synthetic progestin that is used in treating certain neoplasms. It is also approved for the treatment of AIDS patients with diagnosed anorexia, cachexia, or unexplained weight loss. The trade name is Megace.

memory disorder: Any pathological condition affecting mental registration, retention, or recall of past experience, knowledge, ideas, sensations, or thoughts.

meninges: The three membranes that ensheathe the brain and spinal cord: the pia mater (internal), the arachnoid (middle), and the dura mater (external).

meningitis: Inflammation or infection of the membranes of the spinal cord and brain (meninges).

meningoencephalitis: Inflammation or infection of the brain and its meninges.

menses: The monthly flow of bloody fluid from the genital tract of women. *See also* MENSTRUATION.

menstruation: The cyclic discharge of blood and mucosal tissues from the nonpregnant uterus through the vagina. It is brought on by the reduction in production of ovarian hormones, and usually recurs in approximately four-week intervals (pending the lack of pregnancy) in the female during the reproductive period (puberty to menopause). It is the culmination of the menstrual cycle.

mental disorder: Any behavioral or psychological syndrome or pattern typically associated with either a distressing symptom or impairment of function.

meperidine: A narcotic analgesic. The trade name is Demerol.

metabolic acidosis: A disturbance, which results in excessive acid in the body fluids, due to an increase in acids other than carbonic acid. It may be caused by such conditions as severe infection, dehydration, shock, diarrhea, renal dysfunction, or hepatic dysfunction.

metabolic disorder: Any pathological condition that affects the processes, both physical and chemical, by which a substance is handled in the body.

metabolic encephalopathy: Neuropsychiatric disturbances caused by metabolic brain disease. It may be the result of disease in other organs such as the lungs or kidneys; or it may be caused directly by low blood sugar (hypoglycemia), low oxygenation (hypoxia), or decreased blood flow (ischemia).

metastasis: (1) Transfer of a disease, or its manifestations, from one organ or part to another not directly connected with it. (2) Change in location of bacteria or body cells from one part of the body to another.

metastasize: (1) To spread to other parts of the body by metastasis. (2) To form new foci of disease in a distant part of the body by metastasis.

methadone: (1) An agent used to detoxify drug addicts. It is the primary treatment for opiate addiction. (2) An opioid analgesic prescribed to relieve pain. The trade name is Dolophine.

methionine: An essential amino acid. Methionine is a principal supplier of sulfur, which helps prevent disorders of the hair, skin, and nails; helps to lower cholesterol; and helps to reduce fat in the liver and protect the kidneys.

methotrimeprazine: A tranquilizer and analgesic drug. The trade name is Levoprome.

methylphenidate: A drug that is chemically related to amphetamine. In HIV/AIDS patients, methylphenidate has been studied as a treatment for fatigue, AIDS dementia complex, cognitive impairment, and depression. The trade name is Ritalin.

Meticorten: *See* PREDNISONE.

metoclopramide: An antiemetic drug. The trade name is Reglan.

metronidazole: An antiamebic, antibacterial, and antitrichomonal drug appearing as whitish to pale yellowish crystals or crystalline powder. It may be administered orally or intravaginally. The trade name is Flagyl.

microbiology: A branch of biology dealing especially with microscopic forms of life.

Microsporida: An order of parasitic protozoa. *Also called* CNIDOSPORIDIA and MICROSPORIDIA.

Microsporidia: *See* MICROSPORIDA.

microsporidiosis: (1) A pathological condition caused by infection with Microsporidia. (2) An opportunistic infection, caused by Microsporidia, commonly associated with HIV infection. It is recognized as a cause of gastrointestinal disease, sinusitis, renal disease, and keratitis in AIDS patients. Other than general attention to hand washing and other personal hygiene measures, no precautions to reduce exposure can be recommended at this time.

migrating cheilosis: *See* PERLÈCHE.

Military Records Facility: An arm of the National Personnel Records Center from which individuals who have separated from the military may request copies of both their service and health records. Military Records Facility, 9700 Page Avenue, St. Louis, MO 63132-5100. Telephone: (314) 538-4246. Web site, <http://www.nara.gov/regional/stlouis.html>.

milk bank: A facility that collects, pasteurizes, and distributes donor human milk to premature or ill infants and children. The facility may also fill an educational role concerning breast feeding and nutrition.

milzbrand: *See* ANTHRAX.

mineral therapy: Treatment of disease, or pain relief involving the use of minerals.

mineralocorticoid: Any of the biologically active corticosteroids predominantly involved in the regulation of electrolytes and fluid through their effect on ion transport by the renal tubules.

misperception: The state or condition of being perceived incorrectly.

mite: Any arthropod of the order Acarina except ticks. They are minute arachnids related to spiders. Some are parasitic, and are the causative agent of such conditions as mange or scabies. Others serve as intermediate hosts, and carry causative organisms of disease from infected to noninfected individuals.

mitogen: A substance that induces cell division of somatic cells (the cells that become differentiated into the tissues, organs, etc. of the body) in which each daughter cell contains the same number of chromosomes as the parent cell.

molecular biology: A branch of biology dealing with the ultimate physical and chemical organization of living matter, and especially with the molecular basis of inheritance and protein synthesis.

molluscum contagiosum: (1) A viral infection of the skin. (2) A common, mildly contagious, usually self-limited viral infection of the skin characterized by tumor formations on the skin that affects mainly children and young adults. The infection is transmitted by autoinoculation, close contact, and any substance that adheres to and transmits infectious materials. It may also affect adults, and is usually sexually transmitted in this population. The characteristic lesion is a flesh-colored or gray, naval-shaped papule that progresses to pearly white. The core of the papule contains genetic materials surrounded by a protective coat that serves as a vehicle for replication, and may be expelled.

Moniliaceae: A family of colorless to light-colored imperfect fungi belonging to the Moniliases order. These include *Aspergillus, Blastomyces, Coccidioides, Histoplasma, Penicillum, Sporothrix, Trichoderma, Trichophyton, Trichothecium,* and *Verticillium.*

moniliasis: *See* CANDIDIASIS.

monoclonal antibody: (1) An antibody produced for a specific antigen by a hybridoma. (2) Chemically and immunologically homogenous antibodies derived from hybridoma cells. Their exceptional purity and specificity make them useful as laboratory reagents in various tests (e.g., enzyme-linked immunosorbent assay). They are also used experimentally in cancer immunotherapy.

monocyte: (1) A large, mononuclear, nongranular white blood cell. (2) A large, mononuclear, phagocytic leukocyte, with an egg- or kidney-shaped nucleus. They are formed in the bone marrow, and transported to tissues (such as those of the liver or lungs) where they develop into macrophages.

monogamy: Marriage or involvement in an intimate relationship with only one person at a time.

mononucleosis: The presence of an abnormally large quantity of mononuclear leukocytes (monocytes) in the blood. The term is often used to refer to infectious mononucleosis.

monotherapy: Use of only one therapeutic modality, especially drug therapy, to treat an illness or condition.

morbidity: (1) State of being diseased. (2) The number of sick persons or cases of disease in relationship to a specific population.

morphine: The principal alkaloid found in opium, occuring in bitter colorless crystals. Morphine has widespread effects in the central nervous system and on smooth muscle, and is widely used as an analgesic and narcotic. Trade names are MS Contin and Oramorph.

mortality: (1) State of being mortal. (2) The death rate or ratio of number of deaths to a given population.

mortuary science: The science dealing with preparation of the deceased for burial or cremation.

Mothers of AIDS Patients (MAP): Founded in 1985, this organization is divided into local groups that provide support for families of persons with AIDS during the illness and after death. It assists with the formation of local groups, functions as a resource network, and conducts educational presentations. Mothers of AIDS Patients, P.O. Box 3132, San Diego, CA 92013. Telephone: (619) 234-3432.

motor dysfunction: Abnormal, disturbed, or impaired functioning of a muscle, nerve, or center that affects or produces movement.

Motrin: *See* IBUPROFEN.

mourning: The overt expression of grief and bereavement. Mourning is heavily influenced by culture, religion, and society. It includes such practices as donning black or white, attending funerals, crying, and withdrawing from society.

MRI: *See* MAGNETIC RESONANCE IMAGING.

MS Contin: *See* MORPHINE.

mucocutaneous infection: The invasion by and multiplication of a pathogenic agent in a mucous membrane or the skin.

mucosal secretion: (1) The process whereby mucous membranes produce certain materials from the blood. (2) The substances produced by mucous membranes.

mucous membrane: The membrane lining various tubular structures of the body. It consists of a surface layer of epithelium, a basement membrane, and an underlying layer of connective tissue.

mullein: Any of a variety of plants with tall, straight stems, large felty or flannel-like leaves, and long, dense, spiked yellow flowers. The herb is believed to be effective in healing respiratory ailments, asthma, bronchitis, sinus congestion, and useful in treating diarrhea.

multifocal giant-cell encephalitis: *See* AIDS DEMENTIA COMPLEX.

multiple therapy: Use of more than one therapeutic modality, especially drug therapy, to treat an illness or condition.

music therapy: Adjunctive treatment of disease with music. Used especially in cases of neurological, mental, or behavioral disorders.

mutation: (1) A change or transformation. (2) A permanent variation in genetic structure. (3) A change in the genetic material of a gene, which is transmissible to offspring.

mutual masturbation: Reciprocal stimulation of the genitals, or other erogenous zones, for sexual pleasure. The term usually applies to stimulation to the point of orgasm. Mutual masturbation is promoted as a safe sex alternative to penetrative intercourse.

myalgia: Tenderness or pain in a muscle or muscles.

Mycelex G: *See* CLOTRIMAZOLE.

mycobacterial infection: Invasion by and multiplication of *Mycobacterium*. This genus of acid-fast organisms are slender, nonmotile, gram-positive rods that do not produce spores or capsules. It includes the pathogenic causative organisms of tuberculosis and leprosy.

Mycobacterium avium complex: A complex that includes several strains of *Mycobacterium* avium. *Mycobacterium intracellulare* is not easily distinguished from *Mycobacterium avium*, and is therefore included in the complex. These organisms are most frequently found in pulmonary secretions from persons with a tuberculosis-like mycobacteriosis. Strains of the complex have been associated with AIDS as well as childhood lymphadenitis.

Mycobacterium avium-intracellulare **(MAI):** A complex of slow-growing, nonphotochromogenic organisms that are associated with serious systemic disease in AIDS patients, lymphadenitis in children, human pulmonary disease, and cause tuberculosis in birds and swine.

Mycobacterium kansasii: A slow-growing, photochromogenic organism that causes a tuberculosis-like disease in humans.

Mycobacterium leprae: The causative agent of leprosy in humans. They typically occur in rounded masses, groups of bacilli, or intracellular clumps.

Mycobacterium tuberculosis: A slow-growing, nonphotochromogenic, pathogenic organism that causes tuberculosis in humans, primates, hamsters, guinea pigs, and dogs.

Mycobutin: *See* RIFABUTIN.

mycology: The study of fungi.

Mycostatin: *See* NYSTATIN.

myelin: (1) A fat-like substance, composed of lipids and proteins, that coils to form a sheath around the axons of certain nerves, and serves as an electrical insulator. (2) A complex lipoid substance found in small quantities in the brain.

myelitis: (1) Inflammation of the bone marrow. (2) Inflammation of the spinal cord.

myelopathy: (1) A general term denoting any pathological condition of the spinal cord. The term is used to refer to nonspecific lesions as opposed to inflammatory lesions, which are termed myelitis. (2) Any pathological condition of the bone marrow.

myocardial dysfunction: Abnormal, disturbed, or impaired functioning of the muscular tissue of the heart.

myocardial infarction: Condition caused by occlusion of one or more of the coronary arteries. Symptoms include pain or heavy pressure in the center of the chest behind the sternum. Pain may spread to the neck, shoulder, arm, and fourth and fifth fingers of the left hand; to the back, to the teeth, or to the jaw. Nausea and vomiting, sweating, and shortness of breath are also common. Symptoms may come and go. It is imperative that medical care be obtained without delay. *Also called* HEART ATTACK.

myocarditis: (1) Inflammation of the middle layer of the heart wall. (2) Inflammation of the muscular walls of the heart.

myositis: Inflammation of a muscle, especially a voluntary muscle.

mysticism: (1) Any doctrine that asserts the potential of attaining intuitive knowledge of spirituality through meditation. (2) The doctrine that asserts the possibility of communion with God through meditation and contemplation. *See also* MEDITATION.

NAC: *See* CDC NATIONAL AIDS CLEARINGHOUSE.

NAIC: *See* CDC NATIONAL PREVENTION INFORMATION NETWORK.

NAMES Project Foundation: Founded in 1987, this organization was formed to create a patchwork quilt as an appropriate memorial to the AIDS epidemic. Quilt panels are $3' \times 6'$, the size of a human grave. The Foundation seeks to emphasize the humanity of the pandemic, and serves to provide a creative means of expression for those who have been touched by the acquired immunodeficiency syndrome. It produces various publications, raises funds for care of persons with AIDS, and encourages support for infected individuals and their loved ones. Names Project Foundation, 310 Townsend St., Suite 310, San Francisco, CA 94107. Telephone: (415) 882-5500.

NAN: *See* NATIONAL AIDS NETWORK.

Naprosyn: *See* NAPROXE.

naproxen: A nonsteroidal, anti-inflammatory drug used for the treatment of osteoarthritis and rheumatoid arthritis. The trade name is Naprosyn.

NAPWA: *See* NATIONAL ASSOCIATION OF PEOPLE WITH AIDS.

narcotic: A drug, such as opium, that dulls the senses and induces sleep.

nasal ulcer: An open sore or lesion of the nose, accompanied by sloughing of inflamed necrotic tissue.

nasopharynx: The part of the pharynx that lies above the soft palate (postnasal area).

National Academy of Sciences: Founded in 1863, it is an honorary organization that supports the promotion of science and engineering. Members are elected by the Academy in recognition of their contributions to either field. It was founded by an act of Congress to function as the official adviser on scientific and technical matters, and administers the National Academy of Engineering, National Research Council, and Institute of Medicine. National Academy of Sciences, Office of News and Public Information, 2101 Constitution Avenue N.W., Washington, DC 20418. Telephone: (202) 334-2000.

National AIDS Clearinghouse (NAC): *See* CDC NATIONAL PREVENTION INFORMATION NETWORK.

National AIDS Information Clearinghouse (NAIC): *See* CDC NATIONAL PREVENTION INFORMATION NETWORK.

National AIDS Network (NAN): Founded in 1986, this organization—now defunct—was formed to link community-based organizations providing education or direct services to those affected by the acquired immunodeficiency syndrome.

National AIDS Research Foundation: An organization set up in Los Angeles to support AIDS research and disseminate information concerning the disease. It merged with the AIDS Medical Foundation to form the American Foundation for AIDS Research in 1985.

National Archives and Records Administration: The National Archives and Records Administration is charged with assuring ready access to primary sources and other essential evidence that documents the rights of U.S. citizens, the actions of federal officials, and all events pertaining to the national experience. Health and service records of all individuals who have served in either a civilian or military capacity in the federal government, but who are no longer in active service, are available through this agency, as are ship passenger arrival records, census records, land files, military pension records, and a wealth of other information. Researchers may obtain permission to work at the National Archives in Washington, DC, to explore historical documents, images, and realia. National Archives and Records Administration, 700 Pennsylvania Avenue N.W., Washington, DC 20408-0001. Telephone: (800) 234-8861. Web site, <http://www.nara.gov/>.

National Association of People with AIDS (NAPWA): Founded in 1987, it consists of individuals who have tested positive to antibodies indicative of infection with the human immunodeficiency virus, been diagnosed with AIDS-related complex, or developed full-blown AIDS. The Association works to create, implement, and maintain programs throughout the country designed for self-empowerment; promote provision of AIDS-related health care; and expand public understanding of the epidemic. It maintains a speakers' bureau, and provides scholarship and grant funding. National Association of People with AIDS, 1413 K. Street N.W., Washington, DC 20005-3442. Telephone: (202) 898-0414.

National Cancer Institute (NCI): A major component of the National Institutes of Health, NCI is the federal government organization responsible for conducting and supporting cancer research. The Institute oversees a National Cancer Program to expand existing scientific knowledge on cancer cause and prevention as well as the diagnosis, treatment, and rehabilitation of cancer patients. Research activities are carried out in-house or supported through grants or contracts. Cancer research facilities are constructed with Institute support, and training is provided under university-based programs. National Cancer Institute, National Institutes of Health, Building 31, 9000 Rockville Pike, Bethesda, MD 20892. Telephone: (800) 422-6237; TTY: (800) 332-8615. Spanish language materials are available directly from the Web site, <http://nci.nih.gov>.

National Center for Complementary and Alternative Medicine (NCCAM): One of the centers of the National Institutes of Health, NCCAM identifies and evaluates nontraditional health care practices, supports and conducts scientific research on these practices; and disseminates information. Eleven centers across the United States investigate various nontraditional approaches to coping with a variety of health conditions. Three of these centers are particularly relevant to HIV/AIDS: Bastyr University AIDS Research Center, Center for Addiction and Alternative Medicine Research, and the Complementary and Alternative Medicine Program at the University of Texas Center for Alternative Medicine. National Center for Complementry and Alternative Medicine, Clearinghouse, P.O. Box 8218, Silver Spring, MD 20907. Telephone: (888) 644-6226; TTY: (888) 644-6226; Fax: (301) 495-4957. E-mail is available directly from the Web site, <http://nccam.nih.gov>.

National Center for Environmental Health (CEH): One of the nine major components of the Centers for Disease Control, CEH is concerned with the control of environmentally related diseases and chronic diseases. Center for Environmental Health, Centers for Disease Control, Department of Health and Human Services, Public Health Service, 1600 Clifton Road N.E., Atlanta, GA 30333. Telephone: (404) 488-7000.

National Center for Health Statistics (NCHS): Established in 1960 as a division of the Department of Health and Human Services, the Center collects, analyzes, and disseminates national health statistics; administers the Cooperative Health Statistics System; conducts research; organizes and coordinates the efforts of the various Department of Health and Human Services' agencies in health statistics to promote maximum efficiency; cooperates at an international level with organizations concerned with health statistics; and functions as a national resource for health data. It produces various publications and sponsors conferences on health statistics. National Center for Health Statistics, Department of Health and Human Services, Public Health Service, Assistant Secretary for health, 6525 Belcrest Road, Hyattsville, MD 20782. Telephone: (301) 436-7016.

National Center for Infectious Diseases (CID): One of the nine major components of the Centers for Disease Control, CID is concerned with the identification, diagnosis, prevention, and control of infectious diseases. National Center for Infectious Diseases, Centers for Disease Control, Department of Health and Human Services, Public Health Service, 1600 Clifton Road N.E., Atlanta, GA 30333. Telephone: (404) 639-3401.

National Center for Research Resources (NCRR): One of the centers of the National Institutes of Health, NCRR conducts research projects in the areas of biomedical technology, clinical research, comparative medicine, and research infrastructure. National Center for Research Resources, Office of Science Policy, National Institutes of Health, Bethesda, MD 20892. Telephone: (301) 435-0888. E-mail is available directly from the Web site, <http://ncrr.nih.gov/>.

National Commission on AIDS: Created as part of the federal Health Omnibus Programs Extension Act of 1988, the Commission succeeded the Presidential Commission on the Human Immunodeficiency Virus Epidemic. Its purpose is to make recommendations concerning the AIDS epidemic, especially antidiscrimination legislation. *Also called* PRESIDENTIAL COMMISSION ON AIDS.

National Committee to Review Current Procedures for Approval of New Drugs for Cancer and AIDS: The Committee opened in 1989 to review approval procedures for new drugs to be used in the treatment of AIDS and cancer. The parallel track program is an outgrowth of the hearings. *Also called* LASAGNA COMMITTEE HEARINGS. *See also* PARALLEL TRACK.

National Education Association (NEA): Founded in 1857, it is a professional organization and union of elementary and secondary school teachers, college and university faculty, administrators, counselors, principals, and other concerned individuals. The Association produces various publications. National Education Association, 1201 16th Street N.W., Washington, DC 20036. Telephone: (202) 833-4000.

National Endowment for the Arts (NEA): Established in 1965, the NEA invests in the nation's cultural heritage by nurturing the expression of human creativity, supporting the cultivation of community spirit, and fostering the recognition and appreciation of the excellence and diversity in artistic works created by Americans. The NEA has funded many AIDS-related exhibits across the United States. National Endowment for the Arts, 1100 Pennsylvania Avenue N.W., Washington, DC 20506. Telephone: (202) 682-5400. E-mail is available directly from the Web site, <http://www.arts.endow.gov/>.

National Endowment for the Humanities (NEH): The NEH supports learning in history, literature, philosophy, and related areas of the humanities. The foundation funds research, education, museum exhibitions, documentaries, preservation projects, and many activities planned and implemented at the state and local level. National Endowment for the Humanities, 1100 Pennsylvania Avenue N.W., Room 402, Washington, DC 20506. Telephone: (202) 606-8400; Fax: (202) 606-8240. E-mail is available directly from the Web site, <http://www.neh.fed.us/>.

National Eye Institute (NEI): One of the institutes of the National Institutes of Health, NEI both conducts and supports research and training regarding eye diseases that can lead to blindness, visual disorders, visual function, preservation of sight, and all health issues of the blind. NEI also disseminates health information about eye health and blindness. National Eye Institute, 2020 Vision Place, Bethesda, MD 20892. Telephone: (301) 496-5248. E-mail is available directly from the Web site, <http://www.nei.nih.gov/>.

National Gay and Lesbian Task Force (NGLTF): Founded in 1973, this organization is made up of men and women in the United States who are committed to the elimination of prejudice based on sexual orientation. The Task Force offers assistance to individuals and groups working with the homosexual community, produces several publications, and lobbies for gay rights. It was formerly called the National Gay Task Force (NGTF). National Gay and Lesbian Task Force, 2320 17th Street N.W., Washington, DC 20009. Telephone: (202) 332-6483.

National Gay Rights Advocates (NGRA): (Now defunct) Founded in 1978, this public interest law firm was established to promote legal equality for homosexuals. It tried to achieve this goal by bringing cases to court in order to ensure gay and lesbian civil rights in such areas as employment, immigration, and privacy; and it worked to establish legal precedents concerning gay rights. Legal work was free to clients since law firms and attorneys volunteered their services. It operated the AIDS Civil Right Project, which successfully overturned judicial decisions negatively affecting people with AIDS. NGRA produced various publications, and provided legal kits for educational purposes, especially in the areas of couples' rights, trusts, and wills.

National Gay Task Force (NGTF): *See* NATIONAL GAY AND LESBIAN TASK FORCE.

National Heart, Lung, and Blood Institute (NHLBI): One of the institutes of the National Institutes of Health, NHLBI leads a national research program in diseases of the cardiovascular system. NHLBI also conducts a research program into transfusion medicine and supports health education research in these areas. National Institutes of Health, Bethesda, MD 20892. E-mail is available directly from the Web site, <http:www.nhlbi.nih.gov/>.

National Hemophilia Foundation: Founded in 1948, this voluntary organization consists of hemophiliacs, their families, health care professionals, and other concerned individuals. The Foundation sponsors a postgraduate fellowship program to support research, produces various publications, and disseminates information to the public and health care personnel. National Hemophilia Foundation, 116 West 32nd Street, 11th Floor, New York, NY 10001. Telephone: (212) 328-3700.

National Hospice Organization: Founded in 1978, this organization comprises hospice organizations and individuals concerned with the promotion of the hospice concept of care. The Organization works to establish standards of care in the planning and implementation of programs, monitors legislation and regulatory acts concerning hospice care, collects data, conducts educational seminars, sponsors professional and peer group networking, and maintains a nonlending library. National Hospice Organization, 1901 N. Moore Street, Suite 901, Arlington, VA 22209. Telephone: (703) 243-5900.

National Human Genome Research Institute (NHGRI): One of the institutes of the National Institutes of Health, NHGRI supports the NIH component of the Human Genome Project, an international research effort devoted to analyzing the structure of human DNA and to determining the location of the estimated 100,000 human genes. National Institutes of Health, Bethesda, MD 20892. The Director and other key officials can be reached by e-mail directly from the Web site, <http://www.nhgri.nih.gov/>.

National Institute of Allergy and Infectious Diseases (NIAID): Founded in 1948 as a major component of the National Institutes of Health, NIAID conducts and supports broadly based research and research training in the causes, characteristics, prevention, control, and treatment of a wide variety of diseases believed to be attributable to infectious agents (including bacteria, viruses, and parasites), allergies, or other deficiencies and disorders in the responses of the body's immune mechanisms. National Institute of Allergy and Infectious Diseases, National Institutes of Health, Building 31, Room 7A-50, 31 Center Drive MSC 2520, Bethesda, MD 20892. Telephone: (301) 496-5717. E-mail is available directly from the Web site, <http://www.niaid.nih.gov/>.

National Institute of Arthritis and Musculoskeletal and Skin Diseases (NIAMS): One of the institutes of the National Institutes of Health, NIAMS both conducts and sponsors research that investigates the normal structure and function of bones, muscles, and skin, as well as the many diseases that affect these tissues. Epidemiologic studies, research training, and information dissemination represent additional parts of the program. National Institutes of Health, Bethesda, MD 20892. Telephone: (301) 496-8188; Fax: (301) 480-2814. E-mail is available directly from the Web site, <http://www.nih.gov/niams/>.

National Institute of Child Health and Human Development (NICHD): One of the institutes of the National Institutes of Health, NICHD sponsors research on fertility, pregnancy, growth, development, and medical rehabilitation, thereby attempting to assure that all children are born healthy, wanted, and disease-free. National Institute of Child and Human Development, National Institutes of Health, Building 31, Room 2A32, MSC 2425, 31 Center Drive, Bethesda, MD

20892. Telephone: (800) 370-3943; Web site, <http://www.nichdnih. gov/>.

National Institute of Corrections (NIC): The NIC operates through several different centers. The NIC Information Center provides assistance to all correctional agencies—federal, state, and local—that work with adult offenders and provides leadership to influence the development of correctional policies and practices. National Institute of Corrections Administrative Offices, 320 First Street, N.W., Washington, DC 20534. Telephone: (800) 995-6423 or (202) 307-3106. E-mail is available directly from the Web site, <http://199.117.52.250/iinst/>.

National Institute of Dental and Craniofacial Research (NIDCR): One of the institutes of the National Institutes of Health, NIDCR leads a national research program focused on understanding, treating, and preventing both infectious and inherited craniofacial, oral, and dental diseases. National Institute of Dental and Craniofacial Research, National Institutes of Health, Building 31, Room 5B49, MSC 2290, 31 Center Drive, Bethesda, MD 20892. Telephone: (301) 496-4261. E-mail and Spanish language materials are available directly from the Web site, <http://www.nidcr.nih.gov/>.

National Institute of Diabetes and Digestive and Kidney Diseases (NIDDK): One of the institutes of the National Institutes of Health, NIDDK both conducts and sponsors basic and applied research in diabetes and other diseases of the endocrine system and metabolism; nutrition and diseases of the digestive system; diseases of the urinary system; and blood diseases. National Institute of Diabetes and Digestive and Kidney Diseases, Office of Communications and Public Liaison, Building 31, Room 9A04, MSC 2560, 31 Center Drive, Bethesda, MD 20892. Telephone: (301) 496-3583. Both e-mail and Spanish language materials are available directly from the Web site, <http://www.niddk.nih.gov/>.

National Institute of Environmental Health Sciences (NIEHS): One of the institutes of the National Institutes of Health, NIEHS defines how environmental exposures, genetic susceptibility to environmental substances, and age interact to affect individual health. National Institute of Environmental Health Sciences, P.O. Box 12233, Research

Triangle Park, NC 27709. Telephone: (919) 541-3345. E-mail is available directly from the Web site, <http://www.niehs.nih.gov/>.

National Institute of General Medical Sciences (NIGMS): One of the institutes of the National Institutes of Health, NIGMS supports basic biomedical research not focused on specific diseases or disorders. For example, the development of recombinant DNA technology, the basis of the biotechnology industry, was largely the result of research sponsored by NIGMS. National Institute of General Medical Sciences, National Institutes of Health, 45 Center Drive MSC 6200, Bethesda, MD 20892. Telephone: (301) 496-7301. E-mail is available directly from the Web site, <http://www.nigms.nih.gov/>.

National Institute of Justice (NIJ): Founded in 1968, the Institute is the primary Federal sponsor of research on crime and its control, and is a central resource for information on innovative approaches to criminal justice. It sponsors and conducts research, evaluates policies and practices, demonstrates promising new approaches, provides training and technical assistance, assesses new technology for criminal justice, and disseminates its findings at the state and local levels. National Institute of Justice, Department of Justice, 633 Indiana Avenue N.W., Washington, DC 20531. Telephone: (202) 307-2942.

National Institute of Mental Health (NIMH): Founded in 1948, the Institute provides a national focus for the Federal effort to increase knowledge and advance effective strategies to deal with health problems and issues in the promotion of mental health and prevention and treatment of mental illness. It conducts and supports research; provides technical assistance to various organizations; collects, analyzes, and disseminates data; and carries out administrative and financial management function necessary to implement programs. National Institute of Mental Health, Department of Health and Human Services, Public Health Service, 6001 Executive Boulevard, Room 8184, MSC 9663, Bethesda, MD 20892. Telephone: (301) 443-4513; Fax: (301) 443-4279. Key personnel may be reached by e-mail directly from the Web site, <http://www.nimh.nih.gov/>.

National Institute of Neurological Disorders and Stroke (NINDS): One of the institutes of the National Institutes of Health, NINDS supports and conducts research and research training into the basic functions, diseases, prevention, diagnosis, and treatment of disorders and injuries of the nervous system. National Institute of Neurological Disorders and Stroke, Office of Communications and Public Liaison, P.O. Box 5801, Bethesda, MD 20824. E-mail and Spanish language materials are available directly from the Web site, <http://www. ninds.nih.gov/>.

National Institute of Nursing Research (NINR): One of the institutes of the National Institutes of Health, NINR sponsors research programs in which scientists strive to understand and abate the effects of illness and disability, both acute and chronic; promote health behaviors; prevent the onset or exacerbation of disease; and improve the care environment. National Institute of Nursing Research, National Institutes of Health, 31 Center Drive, Room 5B10, MSC 2178, Bethesda, MD 20892. Telephone: (301) 496-0207. E-mail is available directly from the Web site, <http://www.nih.gov/ninr/>.

National Institute on Aging (NIA): One of the institutes of the National Institutes of Health, NIA sponsors research focusing on primary prevention issues in middle-aged and older populations as well as secondary and tertiary prevention of negative behavioral and social consequences of HIV/AIDS. National Institute on Aging, Public Information Office, Building 31, Room 5C27, 31 Center Drive, Bethesda, MD 20892. Telephone: (301) 496-1752. E-mail is available directly from the Web site, <http://www.nih.gov/nia/>.

National Institute on Alcohol Abuse and Alcoholism (NIAAA): One of the institutes of the National Institutes of Health, NIAAA sponsors research focusing on improved methods of treating and preventing alcoholism and related problems in order to reduce the negative consequences of this disease. National Institute on Alcohol Abuse and Alcoholism, National Institutes of Health, 6000 Executive Boulevard, Willco Building, Bethesda, MD 20892. Telephone numbers and e-mail for key personnel are available on the Web site, http://www.niaaa.nih.gov/.

National Institute on Deafness and Other Communication Disorders (NIDCD): One of the institutes of the National Institutes of Health, NIDCD sponsors biomedical research and training relevant to normal functions, diseases, and disorders of hearing, balance, taste, voice, speech, and language. National Institute on Deafness and Other Communication Disorders, Office of Health Communication and Public Liaison, 31 Center Drive MSC 2320, Bethesda, MD 20892. Telephone: (301) 496-7243; TTY: (301) 402-0252; Fax: (301) 402-0018. E-mail is available directly from the Web site, <http://www.nih.gov/nidcd/>.

National Institute on Drug Abuse (NIDA): Founded in 1972, the Institute provides a national focus for the Federal effort to increase knowledge and promote effective strategies in dealing with health problems and issues associated with drug abuse. NIDA conducts and supports research; supports research training and career development; provides technical assistance at various levels; collaborates with organizations and institutions to facilitate and extend programs for the prevention of drug abuse and addiction, and the care, treatment, and rehabilitation of drug abusers; and carries out administrative and financial management functions necessary for the implementation of programs. National Institute on Drug Abuse, Department of Health and Human Services, Public Health Service, Alcohol, Drug Abuse, and Mental Health Administration, 5600 Fishers Lane, Rockville, MD 20857. Telephone: (301) 443-6480. Educational materials are available directly from the Web site, <http://www.nida.nih.gov/>.

National Institutes of Health (NIH): NIH is the primary medical research branch of the federal government, with a mission to improve the health of the American people. To carry out this mission, the agency conducts and supports biomedical research into the causes, prevention, and cure of diseases; supports research training and the development of research resources; and makes use of modern methods to communicate biomedical information. It is organized into the Fogarty International Center, the Clinical Center, the National Library of Medicine, four divisions (Computer Research and Technology, Research Grants, Research Resources, and Research Services), and twelve research institutions (National Cancer Institute; National Heart, Lung, and Blood Institute; National Institute of Arthritis; National Institute of Diabetes, and Digestive and Kidney Diseases; National Institute of Allergy and Infectious Diseases; National Institute of Child Health and Human Development; National Institute of Dental Research; National Institute of Environmental Health Sciences; National Institute of General Medical Sciences; National Institute of Neurological and Communicative Disorders and Stroke; National Eye Institute;

and National Institute on Aging). National Institutes of Health, Department of Health and Human Services, Public Health Service, 9000 Rockville Pike, Bethesda, MD 20892. Telephone: (301) 402-2433. Spanish and English language materials are available directly from the Web site, <http://www.nih.gov/>.

National Labor Relations Board (NLRB): Established in 1935, the NLRB enforces the National Labor Relations Act. Online forms include ways to initiate challenges to labor concerns that include disability questions and health care coverage. National Labor Relations Board, 1099 14th Street N.W., Washington, DC 20570. Complete contact information for local NLRB offices and Spanish language materials are available from the Web site, <http://www.nlrb.gov/>.

National Leadership Coalition on AIDS: Founded in 1987, this organization functions as a clearinghouse concerning AIDS in the workplace. It serves the business and labor communities, while attempting to increase involvement by these groups in the fight against the spread of HIV. The Coalition produces several publications, and maintains an on-site library. National Leadership Coalition on AIDS, 1150 17th Street N.W., Suite 202, Washington, DC 20036. Telephone: (202) 429-0930.

National Lesbian and Gay Health Association (NLGHA): Founded in 1980, this organization comprises health care professionals providing services to homosexuals, and individuals concerned with the quality and availability of care for lesbians and gays. The Association seeks to create, establish, and coordinate interdisciplinary programs and activities to promote a healthier environment for the homosexual community, and to expand the delivery of appropriate care. It promotes and supports research, serves as a liaison at various levels, provides educational services, conducts training programs, compiles statistics, maintains a speakers' bureau, disseminates AIDS information, and sponsors the National Association of People With AIDS. National Lesbian and Gay Health Association, 1407 S. Street N.W., Washington DC, 20009. Telephone: (202) 939-7880.

National Library of Medicine (NLM): The Library, which serves as the Nation's chief medical information source, is authorized to provide medical library services and online bibliographic searching capabilities, such as MEDLINE, AIDSLINE, and others, to public and private agencies and organizations, institutions, and individuals. It is responsible for the development and management of a Biomedical Communications Network, applying advanced technology to the improve, ment of biomedical communications, and operates a computer-based toxicology information system for the scientific community, industry, and other Federal agencies. Through grants and contracts, the Library administers programs of assistance to the Nation's medical libraries that include support of a Regional Medical Library network, research in the field of medical library science, establishment and improvement of the basic library resources, and supporting biomedical scientific publications of a nonprofit nature. National Library of Medicine, National Institutes of Health, Department of Health and Human Services, Public Health Service, 8600 Rockville Pike, Bethesda, MD 20894. Telephone: (301) 594-5983, or toll-free (888) 346-3656; Web site, <http://www.nim.nih.gov/>.

National Minority AIDS Council (NMAC): Founded in 1986, this organization is divided into local, state, and regional groups that *Seek* to address AIDS issues as they affect minority communities, and to support and promote education for minorities. It maintains a speakers' bureau, on-site library, and biographical archives; compiles statistics; produces various publications; and conducts educational and training programs. National Minority AIDS Council, 1931 13th Street N.W., Washington, DC 20009-4432. Telephone: (202) 483-6622.

National Mobilization Against AIDS: Founded in 1984, this organization *Seeks* to increase government funding of AIDS-related services and promote public support of persons with AIDS. It maintains a speakers' bureau for addressing the impact of the AIDS pandemic on civil rights. National Mobilization Against AIDS, 584-B Castro Street, San Francisco, CA 94114-1465. Telephone: (415) 863-4676.

National Personnel Records Center (NPRC): Operated under the auspices of the National Archives and Records Administration, the civilian, military, and health records of all individuals who have served in the federal government are housed in either the Civilian Records Facility or the Military Records Facility. Pension records are housed in Washington, DC. Telephone, fax, and e-mail requests for documents are not accepted, but the proper forms for obtaining the records are easily available from the NPRC's Web site. National Personnel Records Center, Civilian Records Facility, 111 Winnebago Street, St. Louis, MO 63118-4199. Web site, <http://www.nara.gov/regional/stlouis.html>.

National Prevention Information Network: *See* CDC NATIONAL PREVENTION INFORMATION NETWORK.

National Resource Center on Women and AIDS: Founded in 1988, this organization functions as a clearinghouse for issues involving women and AIDS. It conducts research, maintains a speakers' bureau, provides educational and technical support, and produces several publications. National Resource Center on Women and AIDS, 1211 Connecticut Ave N.W., Suite 312, Washington, DC 20036. Telephone: (202) 872-1770.

National Science Foundation (NSF): Established in 1950, the NSF promotes science and engineering through the investment of more that $3.3 billion per year in 20,000 research, development, and education projects. The NSF funds in several areas relevant to HIV/AIDS, including biology, computer and information science, education, and the social and behavioral sciences. National Science Foundation, 4201 Wilson Boulevard, Arlington, VA 22230. Telephone: (703) 306-1234; TDD: (703) 306-0090. E-mail is available directly from the Web site, <http://www.nsf.gov/>.

Native American traditional medicine: A system of medical therapies stemming from the culture and belief system of Native American peoples.

natural killer cells (NK cells): Large, granular lymphocytes that attach themselves to virus-infected cells. The natural killer cells attack and destroy the virus by secreting cytotoxic molecules. They are also effective against some tumor cells. This process is one of the earliest immune defense mechanisms against viral infections.

naturopathy: A therapeutic system that does not use drugs but employs natural forces such as light, heat, water, air, and massage.

NCHS: *See* NATIONAL CENTER FOR HEALTH STATISTICS.

NCI: *See* NATIONAL CANCER INSTITUTE.

NDA: *See* NEW DRUG APPLICATION.

NEA: *See* NATIONAL EDUCATION ASSOCIATION or NATIONAL ENDOWMENT FOR THE ARTS.

NebuPent: *See* AEROSOLIZED PENTAMIDINE.

necropsy: *See* AUTOPSY.

necrosis: (1) The death of areas of tissue. (2) The constellation of morphological changes indicative of cell death, and caused by the progressive degenerative action of various enzymes.

needle cleaning: Use of specific substances (especially bleach) and techniques to render needles reusable, usually for injection drug use by addicts. Needle cleaning has been approved by activists as a mean of reducing HIV transmission in the intravenous drug user community. *See also* NEEDLE-EXCHANGE PROGRAM.

needle sharing: The act, practice, or process of using a hypodermic syringe in common with another or others. Generally the term is applied to drug addicts who reuse a needle after someone else, without sterilizing it, for the purpose of injecting intravenous drugs.

needle-exchange program: Any program established for intravenous drug users educating them or enabling them to exchange used needles and syringes for sterile ones. These programs have been created in an effort to remove contaminated works from this community, and reduce the spread of the human immunodeficiency virus via this route of transmission.

needlestick: The unintentional puncture of the skin with a hypodermic needle.

nef gene: The gene in the human immunodeficiency virus that encodes proteins of 27,000 molecular weight and affects virus replication by decreasing virus production.

negotiation: In the context of HIV/AIDS, refers to discussion between partners, prior to sexual activity, about the practice of safe sex and, perhaps, HIV status.

Neisseria gonorrhoeae: A species of gram-negative bacteria, belonging to the genus *Neisseria,* which cause gonorrhea.

nelfinavir: An HIV protease inhibitor. Nelfinavir was the first protease inhibitor to be made available in a sprinkle formulation for children. The trade name is Viracept.

neonate: (1) A newborn infant. (2) Newly born.

neonatology: Study and care of newborn infants during their first 28 days of life.

neoplasm: Any new and abnormal formation of tissue, such as a growth or tumor. The growth is uncontrolled, progressive, and serves no useful function.

neoplastic: Pertaining to, or of the nature of, a neoplasm; pertaining to new, abnormal, tissue formation.

nephrology: Study of the function and structure of the kidneys.

neurologic complication: A disease or abnormality of the nervous system, which is superimposed upon another disease without being specifically related, yet affecting or modifying the prognosis of the original disease.

neurologic dysfunction: Abnormal, disturbed, or impaired functioning of the nervous system.

neurology: The branch of science dealing with the study of the nervous system and its disorders.

neuropathology: The branch of medicine that deals with the study of diseases of the nervous system, and microscopic and macroscopic structural and functional changes occurring in them.

neuropathy: (1) A general term used to denote pathological changes or dysfunction in the peripheral nervous system. (2) A term used to denote any disease of the nerves.

neuropsychiatric complication: A nervous or mental disease, or difficulty, which is superimposed upon another disease without being specifically related, yet affecting or modifying the prognosis of the original disease.

neuropsychiatry: The branch of medicine concerned with the study of nervous and mental disorders.

neurosurgery: Study and practice of surgically operating on any part of the nervous system.

neurosyphilis: Syphilis affecting the central nervous system. It may be divided into two groups: asymptomatic and symptomatic.

neurotic disorder: *See* MENTAL DISORDER.

Neutrexin: *See* TRIMETREXATE.

neutropenia: A decrease in the number of neutrophil cells in the blood.

neutrophil: (1) A granular leukocyte (white blood cell or corpuscle) with the properties of adherence to immune complexes, chemotaxis, and phagocytosis. They are readily stainable with neutral dyes. (2) Any cell, structure, or histologic element that stains easily with neutral dye.

nevirapine: A non-nucleoside reverse transcriptase inhibitor (NNRTI). Nevirapine is recommended as part of a combination drug therapy to prevent as much replication of HIV in the body as possible. The trade name is Viramune.

New Drug Application (NDA): The status awarded a drug by the Food and Drug Administration that allows it to be sold for profit.

NGLTF: *See* NATIONAL GAY AND LESBIAN TASK FORCE.

NGRA: *See* NATIONAL GAY RIGHTS ADVOCATES.

NGTF: *See* NATIONAL GAY TASK FORCE.

niacin: Part of the vitamin B complex. Niacin protects against pellagra and is essential for proper metabolic functioning of cells.

niacinamide: Part of the vitamin B complex. Niacinamide is used both to prevent and to treat pellagra.

NIAID: *See* NATIONAL INSTITUTE OF ALLERGY AND INFECTIOUS DISEASES.

NIDA: *See* NATIONAL INSTITUTE ON DRUG ABUSE.

night sweat: Profuse sweating at night during sleep. It is often an early sign of disease.

NIH: *See* NATIONAL INSTITUTES OF HEALTH.

Nizoral: *See* KETOCONAZOLE.

NIJ: *See* NATIONAL INSTITUTE OF JUSTICE.

NIMH: *See* NATIONAL INSTITUTE OF MENTAL HEALTH.

NK cells: *See* NATURAL KILLER CELLS.

NLGHA: *See* NATIONAL LESBIAN AND GAY HEALTH ASSOCIATION.

NLM: *See* NATIONAL LIBRARY OF MEDICINE.

NMAC: *See* NATIONAL MINORITY AIDS COUNCIL.

NMRI: *See* MAGNETIC RESONANCE IMAGING.

NNRTI: *See* NON-NUCLEOSIDE REVERSE TRANSCRIPTASE INHIBITOR.

no code: An indication on a terminally ill patient's chart that he/she does not want heroic, life-saving measures or artificial life support when death is imminent. *Also called* NO CODE BLUE or NO CODE-BLUE STATUS. *See also* DURABLE POWER OF ATTORNEY, MEDICAL DIRECTIVE, and LIVING WILL.

no code blue: *See* NO CODE.

no code blue status: *See* NO CODE.

Nocardia: A genus of aerobic, nonmotile actinomycetes that are transitional between bacteria and fungi. Most forms exist on dead organic matter, and some may produce disease in humans.

nocardia: A vernacular term used to denote any member of the genus *Nocardia*.

nocardiosis: An acute or chronic pathological condition caused by infection from any species of *Nocardia*. It may occur as a pulmonary infection, but has a marked tendency to spread to any organ of the body, especially the brain. It results in abscesses in the lungs, brain, skin, or other areas.

node: (1) A knot, knob, protuberance, or swelling. (2) A small mass of tissue in the form of a knot or swelling.

nodular lesion: A circumscribed area of pathologically altered tissue which possesses the characteristics of a nodule.

nodule: A small knot or protuberance that can be detected by touch.

non-Hodgkin's lymphoma: A lymphoma other than Hodgkin's disease. They may be classified into nodular or diffuse tumor patterns and by cell type; or into high, intermediate, and low grade malignancy; and into cytologic subtypes.

non-nucleoside reverse transcriptase inhibitor (NNRTI): Drug that blocks HIV replication by inhibiting the action of the reverse transcriptase enzyme. Nucleoside analogs inhibit the same enzyme, but the two classes of drugs work differently. The NNRTI actually binds with the reverse transcriptase enzyme. *See also* NUCLEOSIDE ANALOG, REVERSE TRANSCRIPTASE, NEVIRAPINE, and DELAVIRDINE.

nonoxynol-9: A spermicide.

nonprogressor: A person who tests positive for HIV antibodies but who remains healthy and does not progress to AIDS.

Norpramin: *See* DESIPRAMINE.

Northern blot technique: A procedure to separate and identify RNA fragments. They are separated by electrophoresis on an agarose gel, blotted onto a nitrocellulose or nylon membrane, and hybridized with labeled nucleic acid probes.

nortriptyline: An antidepressant drug of the tricyclic class. Trade names are Aventyl Hydrochloride and Pamelor.

Norvir: *See* RITONAVIR.

Norwegian scabies: A rare, severe form of scabies characterized by an extremely heavy infestation of mites which appears in patients with poor sensation, severe systemic disease, senility or mental retardation, and immunosuppression.

nosebleed: *See* EPISTAXIS.

NPIN: *See* CDC NATIONAL PREVENTION INFORMATION NETWORK.

nuclear magnetic resonance imaging: *See* MAGNETIC RESONANCE IMAGING.

nucleoside: A glycoside (any of a group of sugar derivatives that when combined with water yields a sugar and one or more other substances) formed by the combination of a sugar (pentose) and a purine or pyrimide base.

nucleoside analog: Drug that blocks HIV from infecting uninfected cells in the body. This class of drug does not help cells that have already been infected. *See also* ZIDOVUDINE, DIDANOSINE, STA-VUDINE, LAMIVUDINE, and ZALCITABINE.

Nuprin: *See* IBUPROFEN.

nutrition: The act or process of nourishing, especially the process by which an individual takes in and utilizes food material.

Nydrazid: *See* ISONIAZID.

nystatin: An antibiotic appearing as a yellowish to tan powder. It is an antifungal used in the treatment of cutaneous, intestinal, oral, or vaginal candidal infections. Nystatin may be administered orally or topically. *Also called* FUNGICIDIN. The trade names are Mycostatin and O-V Statin.

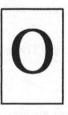

obsessive-compulsive disorder: A condition marked by an inclination to perform certain rituals repetitively in order to relieve anxiety.

occupational exposure: The risk of exposure to a communicable disease through the normal procedures associated with a specific profession (e.g., a needlestick during a surgical procedure).

Occupational Safety and Health Administration (OSHA): Established pursuant to the Occupational Safety and Health Act of 1970, it develops and promulgates occupational safety and health standards; develops and issues regulations; conducts investigations and inspections to determine the status of compliance with regulations; and issues citations and proposes penalties for noncompliance. Occupational Safety and Health Administration, Department of Labor, 200 Constitution Avenue N.W., Washington, DC 20210. Telephone: (202) 693-1999. Web site, <http://www.osha.gov/>.

occupational therapy: Therapeutic use of work, self-care, and play activities to increase independent function, enhance development, and prevent disability.

odynophagia: Pain upon swallowing.

Office of HIV/AIDS Policy: Part of the Office of Public Health and Science that serves under the Surgeon General of the United States, the Office of HIV/AIDS Policy advises the Surgeon General on policy, program, and other issues relevant to HIV. The office also promotes coordination and collaboration with other government entities as well as outside interest groups and community-based organizations. Office of HIV/AIDS Policy, Hubert H. Humphrey Building, Room 730E, 200 Independence Avenue, S.W., Washington, DC 20201. Telephone: (202) 690-5560; Fax: (202) 690-7054; Web site, <http://www.surgeongeneral.gov/ophs.hivaids.htm>.

Office of International and Refugee Health: Part of the Office of Public Health and Science that serves under the Surgeon General of the United States, the Office of International and Refugee Health coordinates participation and cooperation with international bodies as well as agencies within the United States government to provide humanitarian and developmental assistance in health to refugee populations. Office of International and Refugee Health, Parklawn Building, Room 18-75, 5600 Fishers Lane, Rockville, MD 20857. Telephone: (202) 443-1774; Fax: (202) 443-6288; Web site, <http://www.surgeongeneral.gov/ophs/oirh.htm>.

Office of Management and Budget (OMB): Established in 1970 as part of the Executive Office of the President pursuant to Recognition Plan No. 2, the OMB evaluates, formulates, and coordinates management procedures and program objectives within and among federal departments and agencies. It also controls the administration of the federal budget, while routinely providing the President with recommendations regarding budget proposals and relevant legislative enactments. Office of Management and Budget, Executive Office Building, Washington, DC 20503. Telephone: (202) 395-3080. Web site, <http.//www.whitehouse.gov/omb/>.

Office of Minority Health (OMH): Part of the Office of Public Health and Science that serves under the Surgeon General of the United States, the OMH aims to promote and improve health among Native American, Alaska Native, African-American, Asian-American, Pacific Islander, and Hispanic populations in the United States. The office funds grants for health demonstration projects organized by minority community consortia and works cooperatively with seven national minority organizations. Office of Minority Health, Division of Information and Education, Rockwall II Building, Suite 1000, 5600 Fishers Lane, Rockville, MD 20857. Telephone: (301) 443-5224 or toll-free (800) 444-6472; Fax: (301) 443-8280 E-mail is available directly from the Web site, <http://www.omhrc.gov/>.

Office of National AIDS Policy (ONAP): The ONAP provides broad policy guidance and leadership through the White House to direct the federal government's response to the HIV/AIDS pandemic. The Office coordinates White House initiatives and policies with other government agencies as well as external group including community-based organizations. Office of National AIDS Policy, 736 Jackson Place, Washington, DC 20503. Telephone: (202) 456-2437; Fax: (202) 456-2438. E-mail is available directly from the Web site, <http://www.whitehouse.gov/ONAP/>.

Office of National Drug Control Policy: This White House office establishes policies, priorities, and objectives for the federal drug control program, positively affecting three goals: reducing the illicit use, manufacture, and traffic of controlled substances; reducing drug-related crime and violence; and reducing drug-related health problems. Office of National Drug Control Policy, P.O. Box 6000, 2277 Research Blvd., Rockville, MD 20849-6000. Telephone: (800) 666-3332. E-mail is available directly from the Web site, <http://www.white housedrugpolicy.gov/>.

Office of Public Health and Science (OPHS): This office within the Department of Health and Human Services (DHHS) serves as the hub for leadership and coordination throughout the Department in the areas of public health and science; provides direction to all program offices within the OPHS; and provides the Secretary of DHHS advice on public health and science issues as requested. Office of Public Health and Science, Assistant Secretary for Health, U.S. Surgeon General, Hubert H. Humphrey Building, Room 716G, 200 Independence Avenue, S.W., Washington, DC 20201. Telephone: (202) 690-7694; Fax: (202) 690-6960; Web site, <http://www. surgeongeneral.gov/ophs/>.

Office of Science and Technology Policy (OSTP): The OSTP was established in 1976 to provide the President with timely policy advice, and to coordinate the federal government's investment in science and technology. Office of Science and Technology Policy, 1600 Pennsylvania Avenue N.W., Washington, DC 20502. Telephone: (202) 395-7347. E-mail is available directly from the Web site,<http://www.white house.gov/WH/EOP/OSTP/html/OSTP_Home.html>.

Office of Veterans Affairs and Military Liaison: Part of the Office of Public Health and Science that serves under the Surgeon General of the United States, the Office of Veterans Affairs and Military Liaison coordinates health services and information among all uniformed services, the Department of Health and Human Services, the White House, and the National Security Council. The Office provides leadership in resolving health and human service needs of military members, veterans, and their families as well as guiding research that targets sick, disabled, or disadvantaged veterans or active duty military personnel. Office of Veterans Affairs and Military Liaison, Hubert H. Humphrey Building, Room 719H, 200 Independence Avenue, S.W., Washington, DC 20201. Telephone: (202) 260-0576; Web site, <http://www.surgeongeneral.gov/ophs/ovaml.htm>.

Office on Women's Health (OWH): Operated through the U. S. Public Health Service, Department of Health and Human Services, the OWH has developed one of the premier Web sites for women's health. The office works to develop and implement new programs and initiatives to improve the health of women throughout the world; to redress inequities in health research, services, and education that have put women at risk; and to coordinate with other entities, both public and private, that devote themselves to women's health concerns. Office on Women's Health, U.S. Public Health Service, Department of Health and Human Services, 200 Independence Avenue, S.W., Room 730B, Washington, DC 20201. Telephone: (202) 690-7650; Fax: (202) 690-7172. E-mail and Spanish language materials available directly from the Web site, <http://www.4woman.gov/owh/>.

OI: *See* OPPORTUNISTIC INFECTION.

oidiomycosis: *See* CANDIDIASIS.

OMB: *See* OFFICE OF MANAGEMENT AND BUDGET.

Omnipen: *See* AMPICILLIN.

oncogene: A gene found in the chromosomes of tumor cells that has the ability to induce a normal cell to become malignant.

oncogenic: Producing tumors. *See also* PATHOGENIC.

oncology: The study of tumors.

ondansetron: A competitive serotonin type 3 receptor antagonist. It is effective in the treatment of nausea and vomiting caused by cytotoxic chemotherapy drugs. The trade name is Zofran.

oocyst: The encysted form of the fertilized macrogamete, or zygote, in coccidian sporozoa in which sporogonic multiplication occurs. This results in the formation of infectious agents (sporozoites) for the next stage of sporozoan life cycle.

ophthalmology: The science dealing with the eye and its diseases.

opioid: (1) Synthetic narcotics not derived from opium. (2) Indicating substances such as endorphins or enkephalins occurring naturally in the body that act on the brain to decrease the sensation of pain.

opportunistic infection (OI): Invasion and multiplication of microorganisms (especially fungi and bacteria) that under ordinary circumstances do not cause disease, but in certain instances become pathogenic. The infection occurs because the altered physiological state of the host provides the opportunity. In some instances, as when antibiotics are administered over a prolonged period, some microorganisms that ordinarily do not cause disease become pathogenic because of the continued suppression of the more prevalent microorganism. Individuals with impaired immune responses are especially susceptible to opportunistic infections.

oral candida: Candidal infection of the mouth. *See also* CANDIDA.

oral candidiasis: Infection of the skin or mucous membranes in the mouth with any species of Candida. *Also called* PSEUDOMEMBRANOUS CANDIDIASIS and THRUSH. *See also* CANDIDIASIS.

oral herpes simplex: Herpes simplex involving the mouth.

oral lesion: A circumscribed area of pathologically altered tissue or skin in the mouth.

oral leukoplakia: Leukoplakia involving the mouth. *See* HERPES SIMPLEX and LEUCOPLAKIA.

oral sex: Sexual activity in which the genitalia are stimulated with the tongue and mouth.

oral-genital sex: *See* ORAL SEX.

Oramorph: *See* MORPHINE.

Orap: *See* PIMOZIDE.

Orasone: *See* PREDNISONE.

organ bank: An institution that collects, stores, and distributes human organs.

Oriental traditional medicine: A system of traditional medicine that is based on the customs, beliefs, and practices of the Oriental people. Oriental traditional medicine includes Chinese traditional medicine and Kampo medicine. *See also* CHINESE TRADITIONAL MEDICINE and KAMPO MEDICINE.

ornithosis: *See* PSITTACOSIS.

orphan: A child deprived by death of one or usually both parents. No one knows the total number of AIDS orphans, though the Joint United Nations Program on AIDS estimates that by mid-1996, more than 9 million children had lost at least one parent to the pandemic.

orthopedics: The correction or prevention of skeletal deformities.

OSHA: *See* OCCUPATIONAL SAFETY AND HEALTH ADMINISTRATION.

osteopathic medicine: A system of healing that emphasizes manipulation (as of joints) but does not exclude the use of drug therapy and surgery.

otitis media: Inflammation of the middle ear.

otolaryngology: A branch of medicine dealing with the ear, nose, and throat.

otopharyngeal complication: A disease involving the ear and pharynx that is superimposed upon another disease without being specifically related, yet affecting or modifying the prognosis of the original disease.

otorhinolaryngology: *See* OTOLARYNGOLOGY.

O-V Statin: *See* NYSTATIN.

ovine-caprine lentiviruses: Any of the lentiviruses associated with sheep or goats. *See* LENTIVIRUS.

oxidant: An oxidizing agent.

Oxycet: *See* OXYCODONE.

Oxycocet: *See* OXYCODONE.

oxycodone: Semisynthetic derivative of codeine that acts as a narcotic analgesic, and is more potent and addicting than codeine. Trade names are Oxycet, Oxycocet, Ocycontin, Percocet, Roxicodone, Roxilox, and Tylox.

Oxycontin: *See* OXYCODONE.

oxygen therapy: *See* OZONE THERAPY.

ozone therapy: (1) The inhalation of oxygen aimed at restoring toward normal any pathophysiological alterations of gas exchange in the cardiopulmonary system. (2) The inhalation of oxygen in the belief that oxidizing the cells can cure disease.

P

PABA: *See* PARA AMINO BENZOIC ACID.

PAC: *See* PEDIATRIC AIDS COALITION.

pachydermatosis: *See* ELEPHANTIASIS.

paclitaxel: Antineoplastic agent isolated from the bark of the Pacific yew tree, Taxus brevifolia. The trade name is Taxol.

pain: A basic sensation caused by harmful stimuli and marked by discomfort.

pain management: A broad, therapeutic approach to managing physical discomfort.

paleopathology: The study of diseases as found in remains of bodies still extant from ancient times.

palliative care: *See* PAIN MANAGEMENT.

palpation: Application of light fingertip pressure to the outer surface of the body to determine consistency and outline of organs within. *May be part of* PHYSICAL EXAMINATION.

Pamelor: *See* NORTRIPTYLINE.

pancreatitis: Acute or chronic inflammation of the pancreas. It may be symptomatic or asymptomatic; and is most often caused by alcoholism, biliary tract disease, or adverse reaction to the administration of a drug.

pantothenic acid: A vitamin of the B complex group widely distributed in nature, occurring naturally in yeast, salmon, eggs, and various grains; also occurs naturally in the liver and heart.

pap smear: Collection of pooled secretions of the posterior vaginal fornix for cytologic examination. The smear is named for Dr. George Papanicolaou who discovered it. First reported in 1928, its efficacy as a screening tool for the prevention and early detection of cervical cancer was proved by 1941. Widespread use of the pap smear is credited with significant decreases in incidence and mortality from cervical cancer in the developed world. Discovery of the pap smear is widely recognized as the most significant advance in the control of cancer in the twentieth century. *See also* CERVICAL CANCER.

papillary tumor: *See* PAPILLOMA.

papilloma: (1) A benign tumor of the skin or mucous membrane. (2) Any benign epithelial neoplasm. Warts are included in this group. Also called papillary tumor, villoma, and villous papilloma or villous tumor. *See also* PAPILLOMAVIRUS.

Papillomavirus: Any of a group of viruses that cause papillomas in man and animals. They are a subgroup of the papovaviruses.

papovavirus: Any of a group of viruses, many of which are oncogenic (may cause a normal cell to become cancerous), that are important in viral carcinogenesis (cancer-producing). Included in this group are *Papillomaviruses* and *Polyomaviruses*.

papule: A small, circumscribed, elevated, solid, superficial area on the skin.

papulosquamous disease: Any pathological condition of the body characterized by papules and scales such as psoriasis or seborrheic dermatitis.

paraaminobenzoic acid (PABA): A member of the vitamin B complex. It is also employed as a sunscreening agent. The potassium salt is used therapeutically in fibrotic skin disorders.

parallel track: The provision of an alternative track for the administration of experimental drugs to those individuals who do not qualify for clinical trials. This alternative program is an outgrowth of the hearings of the National Committee to Review Current Procedures for Approval of New Drugs for Cancer and AIDS chaired by Louis Lasagna, MD.

parasite: A plant or animal that lives upon, within, or at the expense of another living organism (host) without contributing to that organism's survival. *See also* HOST.

parotiditis: *See* PAROTITIS.

parotitis: Inflammation of the parotid gland. *Also called* PAROTIDITIS.

paroxetine: A serotonin reuptake inhibitor that is effective in the treatment of depression.

paroxysmal: (1) Symptoms occurring in sudden, periodic attacks. (2) Spasmodic, convulsive.

parrot fever: *See* PSITTACOSIS.

partial suppressor: An individual taking highly active antiretroviral therapy (HAART) therapy whose viral load occasionally rises above the undetectable level.

partner: Either individual of a couple dedicated to each other.

partner notification: The act of informing one's sexual partner(s) as to the status of one's health (e.g., divulging the fact that an individual has tested positive to the presence of the human immunodeficiency virus).

passive anal intercourse: *See* RECEPTIVE ANAL INTERCOURSE.

passive immunotherapy: Transfer of immunity from immunized to nonimmune host by administration of serum antibodies or transplantation of lymphocytes.

Pasteur Institute: Founded in 1887, it is considered to be the first institute of large, independent, public hygiene, research organizations. When founded, it served definite practical purposes as well as performing basic research. The Institute currently conducts basic and applied research in biology and medicine including such fields as biochemistry, cellular and molecular biology, developmental biology, immunology, microbiology, mycology, pharmacology, protozoology, and virology. Pasteur Institute, 25-28 Rue du Docteur Roux, 75015 Paris, France. Telephone: +3301 45 68 80 00.

Pasteurella multocida: (1) A bacteria common to the mouth and respiratory tract. (2) A small, nonmotile, gram-negative bacteria that is part of the normal flora of the mouth and respiratory tract of animals and birds. Human disease usually results from an animal bite or scratch, with abscesses, bacteremia, bronchiectasis, localized swelling, meningitis, pneumonia, and septicemia being common symptoms.

patent: (1) An official document open to public examination and granting a certain right or privilege; especially the right to produce, sell, or gain profit from an invention, process, or product for a specified number of years. (2) Produced or sold as a proprietary product. (3) To secure the exclusive right to produce, use, or sell by a patent.

pathogen: Any agent, especially a micro-organism, capable of causing disease.

pathogenesis: (1) The origin and development of a disease. (2) The cellular events and reactions culminating in the development of a disease.

pathogenic: Producing disease. *See also* ONCOGENIC.

pathological: (1) Of pathology. (2) Due to or involving disease.

pathology: (1) The branch of medicine concerned with the nature of disease, especially the functional and structural changes caused by disease. (2) Any conditions, process, or results of a particular disease.

pathophysiology: The study of how normal functions of the living organism and its components are altered by disease.

patient: (1) An individual who is ill, or undergoing treatment for disease or injury. (2) A person receiving medical care.

patient advocacy: Promotion and protection of patients' rights, frequently through a legal process.

patient autonomy: The condition in which the patient maintains control over the direction of his or her treatment.

patient compliance: The degree to which a patient adheres to therapeutic regimens and advice.

patient education: Planned educational activity, generated by a health professional and conducted through clinician review. The goal of patient education is to convey knowledge, attitudes, and skills with the express aim of changing behavior or increasing compliance with therapy in order to improve health and quality of life.

patient zero: The individual suspected of being the first person with AIDS responsible for infiltrating a country and promoting the spread of the disease among its inhabitants.

Paxil: *See* PAROXETINE.

PCP: *See* PNEUMOCYSTIS CARINII PNEUMONIA.

PCR: *See* POLYMERASE CHAIN REACTION.

pediatric AIDS: The condition involving the acquired immunodeficiency syndrome in individuals between birth and the age of 13. *See also* ACQUIRED IMMUNODEFICIENCY SYNDROME.

Pediatric AIDS Coalition (PAC): This advocacy group seeks to promote AIDS treatment, research, and education for children. Pediatric AIDS Coalition, 1331 Pennsylvania Avenue N.W., Suite 721-N, Washington, DC 20004. Telephone: (202) 662-7460.

pediatrics: A branch of medicine dealing with the care and diseases of children.

peer education: The action or process of educating individuals of equal standing.

peliosis hepatis: A condition characterized by blue patches on the liver. It is caused by blood-filled spaces in those parts of the liver that are concerned with its function rather than its structure.

pellagra: Disease or syndrome caused by a deficiency of niacin or by the body's failure properly to absorb niacin from the diet. Symptoms may manifest themselves on the skin, in the gastrointestinal system, or in the nervous system.

pelvic inflammatory disease (PID): Inflammation in the pelvic cavity. It may be acute or chronic, and often involves pus-forming lesions in the female genital tract.

pemoline: A central nervous system stimulating drug. The trade name is Cylert.

penicillin: A large group of antibacterial antibiotics that are biosynthesized by several species of molds of the genus *Penicillium*. Produced naturally as well as synthetically, penicillin is especially effective on gram-positive bacteria as well as on certain gram-negative pathogens.

Penicillium: A genus of fungi, with certain species yielding antibiotic substances and biologicals (e.g., *Penicillium chrysogenum* yields penicillin).

Pension and Welfare Benefits Administration (PWBA): An agency operating under the Department of Labor, PWBA is responsible for protecting the integrity of pensions, health plans, and other employee benefits for workers in the United States. U.S. Department of Labor, PWBA Office of Public Affairs, 200 Constitution Avenue, N.W., Room N-5656, Washington, DC 20210. Telephone: (202) 219-8921. Spanish language materials are available directly from the Web site, <http://www.dol.gov/dol/pwba/>.

pentafuside: Generic name for an antiretroviral, fusion inhibitor drug.

pentamidine: A drug used in the treatment of pneumonia due to *Pneumocystis carinii. See also* AEROSOLIZED PENTAMIDINE and PENTAMIDINE ISETHIONATE.

pentamidine isethionate: A toxic drug effective in the treatment of *Pneumocystis carinii* pneumonia; and also used in the prophylaxis and treatment of early stages of African sleeping sickness. Since it does not cross the blood-brain barrier, it is not effective in the advanced stage of this disease.

Pentatrichomonas hominis: A species of parasitic protozoan flagellates, belonging to the genus *Pentatrichomonas* that live as a commensal in the colon of humans and a variety of animals. Formerly called *Trichomonas hominis*.

pentose: A monosaccharide (a carbohydrate not decomposable by hydrolysis) containing five carbon atoms in the molecule (e.g., arabinose, ribose).

People with AIDS Coalition: Founded in 1985, the Coalition comprises local support networks for person with AIDS. It conducts research, operates a speakers' bureau, maintains a library, produces various publications, serves as a liaison to social service organizations, and operates a drop-in service. People with AIDS Coalition, 50 W. 17th Street, 8th Floor, New York, NY 10011-1607. Telephone: (212) 647-1415.

peptide T: A small polypeptide (a substance containing two or more amino acids in the molecule joined together by peptide linkages) that has been reported, in the laboratory, to block the binding of HIV to the surface of susceptible cells. Research is in progress to confirm the in vitro studies; and an investigational new drug status has been granted by the Food and Drug Administration allowing for Phase I clinical trials.

Percocet: *See* OXYCODONE.

percussion: Act of lightly striking part of the body with short, sharp blows to aid in diagnosing a condition beneath the sound heard. May be part of PHYSICAL EXAMINATION.

percutaneous: Performed through the skin (e.g., injection or removal accomplished by a needle inserted through the skin).

pericarditis: Inflammation of the pericardium (the outside lining of the heart).

pericardium: The fibroserous sac enclosing the heart and the origins of the great blood vessels. It consists of an inner serous layer (epicardium or visceral pericardium) and an outer layer of fibrous tissue (parietal pericardium). The base of the pericardium is attached to the diaphragm.

perinatal: The period shortly before and after birth. It ranges in definition from the twenty-eighth week of pregnancy through 7 days after birth in its shortest form, to the twentieth week of gestation through 28 days after birth in its longest form.

perinatal transmission: Vertical transmission of HIV from mother to fetus or neonate during the perinatal period.

periodontal disease: Any pathologic condition of the supporting structures of the teeth (periodontium).

periodontitis: Inflammation or degeneration, or both, of the dental periosteum, alveolar bone, cementum, and adjacent gingiva.

peritoneal cavity: A potential space between layers of the parietal and visceral peritoneum.

peritoneal dialysis: Dialysis in which the lining of the peritoneal cavity is used as the dialysis membrane. The dialyzing solution is introduced into and removed from the peritoneal cavity.

peritoneum: The serous membrane reflected over the viscera and lining the abdominopelvic walls.

peritonitis: Inflammation or infection of the peritoneum. It is accompanied by abdominal pain, constipation, vomiting, and fever.

perlèche: A disorder marked by single or multiple fissures and cracks at the corners of the mouth. In advanced stages, it may spread to the lips and cheeks. It may be due to oral candidiasis, a dietary deficiency, poor hygiene, drooling of saliva, or other causes. *Also called* ANGULAR CHEILITIS, ANGULAR CHEILOSIS, ANGULAR STOMATITIS, MIGRATING CHEILOSIS, and INTERTRIGO LABIALIS.

persistent generalized lymphadenopathy (PGL): Lymph node enlargement of 1 centimeter or greater at two or more extrainguinal sites, and persisting for more than three months without a concurrent illness, condition, or any explanation other than infection with the human immunodeficiency virus. PGL constitutes Group III of the Centers for Disease Control's classification system for HIV infection.

person with AIDS (PWA): An individual diagnosed with the acquired immunodeficiency syndrome.

person with AIDS-related complex (PWARC): An individual diagnosed with AIDS-related complex, a precursor to the acquired immunodeficiency syndrome.

personal hygiene: (1) An individual's practices used for the preservation of health and prevention of disease. (2) Cleanliness, sanitary practices.

perspiration: (1) Sweat. (2) Salty fluid secreted through the sweat glands of the skin.

Pertofrane: *See* DESIPRAMINE.

PET scan: *See* POSITRON EMISSION TOMOGRAPHY.

PGL: *See* PERSISTENT GENERALIZED LYMPHADENOPATHY.

PHA: *See* PHYTOHEMAGGLUTININ.

phagocyte: Any cell that ingests and destroys other cells, microorganisms, or other foreign matter in the blood or tissues.

phagocytosis: The process of cells engulfing, ingesting, and digesting solid substances such as bacteria, other cells, or foreign particles.

pharmacological therapy: The use of drugs to prevent or treat disease.

pharmacology: The branch of science dealing with the study of the origin, nature, properties, uses, and effects of drugs.

phenothiazine: An organic compound used in manufacturing a certain class of tranquilizers.

phenylalanine: An essential amino acid formed from protein.

phosphatidylcholine: Derivative of phosphatic acid in which the phosphoric acid is bound in ester linkage to a choline moiety.

phosphonoformate: *See* FOSCARNET.

photosensitivity disorder: Abnormal reaction to light, especially sunrays or ultraviolet light.

PHT: *See* PASSIVE HYPERIMMUNE THERAPY.

physical examination: Examination of the body by auscultation, palpation, percussion, inspection, and smelling.

physical therapy: Rehabilitation related to restoration of function and prevention of disability following disease, injury, or loss of body part.

physician assistant: A specially trained (and licensed when necessary) individual who performs tasks usually done by a physician under the direction of a supervising physician.

physiology: A science dealing with the functions and functioning of living matter and beings.

phytohemagglutinin (PHA): A lectin found in the red kidney bean that agglutinates (joins by adhesion) erythrocytes and stimulates predominantly T lymphocytes.

phytotherapy: *See* HERBAL MEDICINE.

PI: *See* PROJECT INFORM or PRINCIPAL INVESTIGATOR.

PID: *See* PELVIC INFLAMMATORY DISEASE.

pimozide: An antipsychotic agent. Also used for the suppression of vocal and motor tics in patients with Tourette's syndrome. The trade name is Orap.

pine bark extract: A nutrient believed to be an effective antioxidant. *Also called* PYCNOGENOL.

pinocytosis: The cellular process of actively engulfing liquid.

piritrexim: (1) A folic acid antagonist. (2) A lipid-soluble antifolate shown to have activity against both *Pneumocystis carinii* and *Toxoplasma gondii*. Studies are currently under way to judge the effectiveness of this drug.

Pitressin: *See* VASOPRESSIN.

placebo: An inactive substance with no medical value. Initially administered for the sole purpose of satisfying a patient's psychophysiological craving for medication; more recently, placebos have been administered to the control group (of a controlled clinical trial) in order to distinguish the effects of the experimental treatment. *See also* CONTROL GROUP and CLINICAL TRIAL.

plasmacytosis: An excess of plasma cells in the blood.

plasmapheresis: The separation of the cellular elements of the blood from the plasma, after it has been withdrawn from the body. The packed red cells are then retransfused into the donor, or to an individual requiring red cells rather than whole blood.

platelet: A round or oval disk found in the blood of vertebrates.

play therapy: Involvement in sport, amusement, or recreation for therapeutic use.

PLWA: *See* PERSON WITH AIDS.

PML: *See* PROGRESSIVE MULTIFOCAL LEUKOENCEPHALOPATHY.

pneumococcal vaccine: A vaccine that induces immunity against certain capsule types of disease caused by the pneumococcus bacterium.

pneumococcus: An oval-shaped, encapsulated, nonspore-forming, gram-positive organism causing such infections as pneumonia, mastoiditis, otitis media, bronchitis, meningitis, keratitis, bloodstream infections, and conjunctivitis.

Pneumocystis carinii: (1) The causative agent of *Pneumocystis carinii* pneumonia. (2) A genus of microorganisms that cause the acute interstitial cell pneumonia, *Pneumocystis carinii* pneumonia.

Pneumocystis carinii **pneumonia (PCP):** Protozoal infection of the pulmonary system that generally presents symptoms of fever, cough, difficulty or pain in breathing, and tightness of the chest. Trimethoprim-sulfamethoxazole and pentamidine isethionate are both used as standard drug therapies.

pneumonia: Inflammation of the lungs caused primarily by bacteria, chemical irritants, and viruses, and resulting in solidification of the lung tissue.

pneumonitis: Inflammation of the lungs. *See also* PNEUMONIA.

podiatry: The care and treatment of the human foot.

podophyllotoxin: A highly toxic compound that has cathartic and antineoplastic properties.

poetry therapy: Use of poems or metrical writing for therapeutic use.

pol gene: The gene that encodes the reverse transcriptase enzyme of the human immunodeficiency virus, transcribes viral RNA into DNA, and encodes a portion of the HIV protease and an endonuclease protein.

poliomyelitis vaccine: *See* POLIOVIRUS VACCINE INACTIVATED.

poliovirus vaccine inactivated (IPV): A suspension of three types of inactivated poliovirus (I, II, III) used both in the immunization of unimmunized adults and for immunologically deficient patients. *Also called* POLIOMYELITIS VACCINE and SALK VACCINE.

Polycillin: *See* AMPICILLIN.

polymerase chain reaction (PCR): In vitro method for producing large amounts of specific DNA or RNA fragments of defined length and sequence from small amounts of short, oligonucleotide-flanking sequences (primers). The essential steps include thermal denaturation of the double-stranded target molecules, annealing of the primers to their complementary sequences, and extension of the annealed primers by enzymatic synthesis with DNA polymerase. The reaction is efficient, specific, and extremely sensitive. Uses for the reaction include disease diagnosis, detection of difficult-to-isolate pathogens, mutation analysis, genetic testing, DNA sequencing, and analysis of evolutionary relationships.

Polymox: *See* AMOXICILLIN.

polyneuropathy: A disease that involves a number of nerves.

polyomavirus: Any of a subgroup of the papovaviruses that causes malignancies in lower animals (e.g., mice).

polyprotein: Nitrogenous, organic compound, containing more than about 100 amino acid residues, in vegetable and animal matter. Proteins yield amino acids on hydrolysis, and are foods assimilated as amino acids and reconstructed in the protoplasm.

poppers: *See* AMYL NITRITE INHALANT and BUTYL NITRITE INHALANT.

porphyria: Any of a group of disturbances in porphyrin metabolism, characterized by increased formation and excretion of porphyrins or their precursors.

porphyrin: Any of a group of nitrogen-containing organic compounds, obtained from chlorophyll and hemoglobin, that occur in protoplasm and form the basis of respiratory pigments in plants and animals.

positron emission tomography (PET scan): A procedure that produces transverse sectional images of the body by the demonstration of the internal distribution of positron-emitting radionuclides.

postmortem examination: *See* AUTOPSY.

postpartum: Occurring after childbirth or delivery. The term refers to the mother.

post-traumatic stress disorder (PTSD): The development of characteristic symptoms after a psychologically traumatic event generally outside the range of usual human experience. Symptoms vary from individual to individual.

postural hypotension: A decrease in blood pressure upon rising to an erect position or posture. Although normal, it may cause fainting under certain conditions (e.g., rising after having been bedridden for several days). *See also* BLACKOUT and SYNCOPE.

potassium: Mineral element found in combination with other elements in the body.

power of attorney: A written statement legally authorizing a person to act on behalf of another. *See also* DURABLE POWER OF ATTORNEY.

practice guideline: A set of directions or principles presenting current or future rules of policy for the health care practitioner. Guidelines are designed to assist in patient care decisions regarding diagnosis, treatment, or related clinical circumstances.

pre-cum: *See* PRE-EJACULATORY SECRETION.

prednisone: A steroid hormone derived from cortisone. It is administered orally to treat various conditions which respond to the anti-inflammatory properties of this type of hormone. Also called delta-cortisone. The trade names are Deltasone, Meticorten, Orasone, and SK-Prednisone.

pre-ejaculatory secretion: The ejection of semen prior to orgasm.

prejudice: (1) An opinion for or against something without adequate basis. (2) To damage by judgement or action.

premarital testing: Testing prior to marriage for the presence of antibodies indicative of specific diseases.

prepartum: Occurring just before childbirth. The term refers to the mother.

Presidential Commission on AIDS: *See* PRESIDENTIAL COMMISSION ON THE HUMAN IMMUNODEFICIENCY VIRUS EPIDEMIC and NATIONAL COMMISSION ON AIDS.

Presidential Commission on the Human Immunodeficiency Virus Epidemic: Established by President Reagan in 1987, the Commission was founded to make recommendations at the federal level concerning the HIV epidemic, especially antidiscrimination legislation. It was succeeded in 1988 by the National Commission on AIDS. *Also called* PRESIDENTIAL COMMISSION ON AIDS and WATKINS COMMISSION.

presumptive diagnosis: (1) A diagnosis based on reasonable grounds for conclusions established by previous, and commonly accepted, experience. This procedure may be used when diagnostic tests are not available or cannot be obtained. (2) The opposite of definitive diagnosis.

prevalence: The number of cases of a disease present in a population at a specific point in time. *See also* INCIDENCE.

primary care: Basic or general health care provided at the person's first contact with the health care system. Generally deemed sufficient for common illnesses.

Princeton rub: *See* FROTTAGE.

principal investigator (PI): The director of a research project that is either partially or fully supported by grant funding.

Principen: *See* AMPICILLIN.

prochlorperazine: A phenothiazine-type drug used in treating nausea and vomiting. The trade name is Compazine.

Procrit: *See* ERYTHROPOIETIN.

proctitis: Inflammation of the anus and rectum. Blood, mucus, or pus may be present in the excrement.

proctocolitis: Inflammation of the colon and rectum. *Also called* COLOPROCTITIS.

proctology: Phase of medicine dealing with treatment of diseases of the colon, rectum, and anus.

prognosis: The forecast or prediction as to the course and outcome of a disease. Also the estimate of recovery from a disease based on the conditions exhibited by the case.

progressive multifocal leukoencephalopathy (PML): A disease in which destruction of the myelin sheath of the nerve is usually found in the white matter of the brain, but it is rarely found in the brain stem and cerebellum. It occurs secondary to various neoplastic diseases, and is generally fatal.

Project Inform (PI): Founded in 1985, it was established to disseminate information concerning experimental treatments for the acquired immunodeficiency syndrome or the human immunodeficiency virus, and to lobby for expanded research and health care services in this area. Project Inform produces an information packet of materials. Project Inform, 1965 Market Street, Suite 220, San Francisco, CA 94103. Telephone: (415) 558-8669.

proline: An important amino acid formed by decomposition of protein.

promiscuity: (1) The state, quality, or instance of exercising a lack of discrimination, specifically with reference to engaging in sexual activities. (2) The state, quality, or instance of casually engaging in sexual intercourse with one or more people.

prophylaxis: The prevention of disease; treatment to prevent disease.

propolis: A sticky resin present in the buds and bark of certain trees and plants. It is collected by bees for the purpose of repairing combs, filling cracks, and waterproofing the hive. There is anecdotal evidence that propolis may be effective in treating certain diseases.

propoxyphene: A narcotic analgesic structurally related to methadone. Trade names are Darvon, Dolene, and SK65.

prostitute: A man or woman who engages in promiscuous heterosexual or homosexual sexual intercourse for pay. *Also called* HOOKER.

protease inhibitor: A compound that inhibits or antagonizes biosynthesis or actions of protease.

protease paunch: Side effect of some protease inhibitors in which a layer of fat tissue gathers around the midsection of the body, particularly the abdomen. The side effect was not reported in initial clinical trials but appears to occur following longer-term use of the drugs.

protein: One of a class of complex nitrogenous compounds that occur naturally in plants and animals, and yield amino acids when hydrolyzed. Proteins provide the amino acids necessary for the growth and repair of animal and human tissue.

protocol: A detailed plan for the conduct of an experiment.

Protozoa: The subkingdom that includes the simplest organisms of the animal kingdom. It consists of unicellular organisms that range in size from submicroscopic to macroscopic. Reproduction is usually asexual by fission, but conjugation and sexual reproduction do occur. Most are free living, but some exist as commensals, mutualists, or parasites.

protozoal infection: The state or condition in which the body is invaded by Protozoa.

protozoan: (1) Concerning or pertaining to Protozoa. (2) An individual of the Protozoa.

provirus: The precursor of a virus.

Prozac: *See* FLUOXETINE.

pruritic papule: A pale, dome-shaped, intensely itchy lesion with a small vesicle on top that progresses to crusting.

pseudomembranous candidiasis: *See* ORAL CANDIDIASIS.

psittacosis: An acute or chronic respiratory and systemic infectious disease that is caused by *Chlamydia psittaci*. Although it affects primarily parrots and other birds, it may be transmitted to humans. Human infection is generally caused by inhaling dried, contaminated bird excreta, or occasionally by handling bird products containing the pathogen. Infection may be asymptomatic. When symptoms appear, they range from a mild influenza-like manifestation to a severe and fatal pneumonia. *Also called* ORNITHOSIS and PARROT FEVER.

psoriasis: (1) A chronic skin disease characterized by scaley, reddish patches. (2) A common, autoimmune, chronic, inflammatory disease of the skin characterized by flare-ups and remissions, and consisting of erythematous papules that come together to form plaques with distinct borders. It has an affinity for the extensor surfaces, genitalia, lumbosacral region, nails, and scalp. If the disease is untreated and progression continues, silvery to yellow-white scales may develop. Severity of the disease ranges from a minimal cosmetic problem to total body involvement and sometimes can be life threatening (psoriatic erythroderma).

psychiatry: The branch of medicine that deals with diagnosis, treatment, and prevention of mental illness.

psychoanalysis: Methods of obtaining a detailed account of past and present mental and emotional experience and repressions in order to determine the source, and to eliminate or diminish the undesirable effects of unconscious conflicts by making the patient aware of their existence, origin, and inappropriate expression in emotions and behavior.

psychology: The science dealing with mental processes, both normal and abnormal.

psychoneuroimmunology: The field concerned with the interrelationship between the brain, behavior, and the immune system.

psychosis: A mental disorder characterized by personality disintegration, and gross impairment of perception and contact with reality. The disturbances are generally marked by delusions, hallucinations, and incoherent speech. The term may also be applied, in a more general sense, to refer to disorders in which impaired mental functioning results in an interference with the patient's ability to cope with the daily demands of life.

psychosocial issue: A result, consequence, or outcome relating to both psychological and social factors.

pteroylglutamic acid: *See* FOLIC ACID.

PTSD: *See* POST-TRAUMATIC STRESS DISORDER.

Public Health Service (PHS): The office of the U.S. Surgeon General, the National Institutes of Health, the Centers for Disease Control and Prevention, the Food and Drug Administration, the Indian Health Service, and many other federal government office and agencies, fall under the administration of the PHS. PHS is a uniformed agency of the federal government. Web site, <http://phs.os.dhhs.gov/phs.phs.html>.

pulmonary alveolar proteinosis: A chronic lung disease of unknown cause in which eosinophilic material is deposited in the alveoli. This prevents ventilation of the affected areas. It is characterized by dyspnea (shortness of breath or difficulty in breathing), chest pain, weakness, and weight loss. Pulmonary insufficiency may lead to death.

pulmonary dysfunction: Abnormal, disturbed, or impaired functioning of the lungs.

pulmonology: The study of the respiratory system.

purine: A colorless, crystalline, heterocyclic compound that is the parent compound of purine bases (e.g., adenine, caffeine, guanine, uric acid, and xanthine).

purpura: A small hemorrhage (up to 1 centimeter in diameter) in the skin, mucous membranes, internal organs, and other tissues resulting from varied causes including blood disorders, trauma, and vascular abnormalities.

PWA: *See* PERSON WITH AIDS.

PWARC: *See* PERSON WITH AIDS-RELATED COMPLEX.

pycnogenol: *See* PINE BARK EXTRACT.

pyridoxine: *See* VITAMIN B-6.

pyrimethamine: An antiviral drug appearing as a white crystalline powder. It is used in the prophylaxis of malaria, and also in conjunction with a sulfonamide in the treatment of toxoplasmosis. Pyrimethamine is administered orally. The trade name is Daraprim.

pyrimethamine/sulfadiazine: Combined drug therapy using pyrimethamine and sulfadiazine.

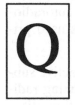

Qi: The virtual life force in the body, supposedly conducive to regulation by acupuncture.

quality of life: A concept that differs for each person, and may vary for the same individual as that person's life situation changes. The goal is to have the quality of life be as good as possible under existing circumstances.

quarantine: (1) Any isolation or restriction of movement imposed on apparently well individuals after having been exposed to an infectious disease in an effort to control its spread. (2) The period of detention at entering a country (originally 40 days). (3) The period of isolation following the onset of contagious disease. (4) The place where individuals are detained for observation.

radiation therapy: (1) Treatment of disease by radiation. (2) One of three major treatment modalities for some types of cancer. The goal of radiation therapy is to minimize damage to healthy tissue surrounding a diseased area, while at the same time delivering a dose of ionizing radiation powerful enough to diminish or destroy the malignant cells. Usually, radiation therapy for cancer patients is delivered either through teletherapy (radiation source is outside the body) or brachytherapy (radiation source is implanted inside the body).

radiography: The making of film images (filming) of the internal structure of the body through exposure to x-radiation, which acts on a sensitized film.

radioimmunoassay (RIA): A highly sensitive method of determining the concentration of substances achieved by using the competition between radioactively labeled hormones and specific antibodies. It can be used to determine the concentration of protein-bound hormones in blood plasma, any substance which causes the production of a specific antibody, or antibody concentrations.

radioimmunoprecipitation assay (RIPA): A method of HIV antibody testing in which the virus is detected by the phenomenon of aggregation of sensitized antigen upon addition of specific antibody to antigen in solution (immunoprecipitation). The precipitate is then washed extensively, and disrupted and distributed through a polyacrylamide gel. Antibody-antigen bands are detected by autoradiography. The technique is technically demanding, and is used primarily in research.

radiology: The branch of medicine concerned with radioactive substances, including X rays, radioactive isotopes, and ionizing radiations, and the application of this information to prevention, diagnosis, and treatment of disease.

radiotherapy: The treatment of disease by the application of radiation.

randomized controlled trial: An experimental study for assessing the effects of a particular variable (such as treatment or drug) in which subjects are assigned on a random basis to either of two groups, experimental or control. The experimental group receives the drug or procedure, while the control group does not.

rape: Sexual intercourse (heterosexual or homosexual) that occurs against the will of the victim.

rapid progressor: HIV-infected individual who progresses to AIDS more quickly than the majority of cases, which typically, historically, have been 7 to 10 years.

receptive anal intercourse: Sexual intercourse in which an individual allows the insertion of a penis into his or her anus. This is a highly efficient mode of transmission for the human immunodeficiency virus. *Also called* PASSIVE ANAL INTERCOURSE.

rectal douche: A current or stream of water directed against the rectum. It may be plain or medicated water.

rectal mucosa: A mucous membrane that lines the rectum.

rectum: The lower portion of the large intestine that is located between the sigmoid flexure and the anal canal.

red blood cell: *See* ERYTHROCYTE.

red blood corpuscle: *See* ERYTHROCYTE.

reflexology: Study of reflexes.

refractory: Recurring; not yielding to treatment.

Reglan: *See* METOCLOPRAMINDE.

rehabilitation therapy: The process of treatment and education that leads the disabled individual to attain maximum function, a sense of well-being, and a personally satisfying level of independence.

Reiki massage: A form of massage in which higher vibrations of energy are channeled through the individual's auric field and into the body. The goal is to harmonize and bring balance to the total self.

Reiter's syndrome: A triad of symptoms consisting of arthritis, conjunctivitis, and urethritis; urethritis generally appears first, but arthritis constitutes the dominant feature. The syndrome is of unknown etiology, and generally runs a self-limited but relapsing course.

relapse: Recurrence of disease or symptoms after apparent recovery.

remission: (1) Abatement or diminution of the symptoms of a disease. (2) The period of time during which abatement or diminution of the symptoms of a disease occurs.

replication cycle: The process of duplication of genetic material.

Rescriptor: *See* DELAVIRDINE.

respirator: (1) An apparatus or machine that can be used to artificially control ventilation. (2) A device that assists with pulmonary ventilation. (3) A mechanical method of filtering the air inhaled through it.

respiratory alkalosis: A metabolic condition resulting from an excessive loss of carbon dioxide from the lungs.

respiratory distress syndrome: Severe impairment of the function of respiration.

respiratory therapy: Treatment to preserve or improve pulmonary function.

resuscitation: The restoration or revival of vital signs of life after apparent death.

reticuloendothelial cell: (1) A phagocytic cell of the reticuloendothelial system. (2) A cell possessing the ability to isolate and ingest inert particles and vital dyes.

reticulosis: An abnormal increase in the number of cells related to reticuloendothelial cells.

retina: The innermost of three tunics of the eye. It receives images formed by the lens as light rays come to focus on the light-sensitive structure. The retina extends from the anterior entrance point of the optic nerve to the pupil. It is comprised of three parts: pars optica (the nervous or sensory portion that extends from the optic disk to the ora serrata, resting behind the ciliary process); pars ciliaris (the portion that lines the ciliary process); and pars iridica (the portion which rests on the posterior surface of the iris). The macula lutea, the most sensitive part of the retina, lies in the posterior portion of the retina. In the center of the macula lutea lies the depression called the fovea centralis. This is the region of most acute vision. Inside the fovea centralis is the point at which nerve fibers exit the retina to form the optic nerve. This point is called the optic papilla, and is devoid of rods and cones, leaving it insensitive to light. From without, the retina is composed of pars pigmentosa (an outer pigment epithelium) and pars nervosa, which consists of nine layers (a layer of rods and cones, the external limiting membrane, the outer nuclear layer, the outer plexiform layer, the inner nuclear layer, the inner plexiform layer, the layer of ganglion cells, the nerve fiber layer, and the internal limiting membrane).

retinitis: Inflammation of the retina.

retinochoroiditis: *See* CHORIORETINITIS.

Retrovir: *See* ZIDOVUDINE.

retrovirus: The common name for the large family of RNA viruses which carry reverse transcriptase. These include the lentiviruses and leukoviruses.

rev gene: The gene in the human immunodeficiency virus, which is required for viral protein RNA processing.

reverse transcriptase: Any enzyme that catalyzes the process of forming a compound, by combining simpler molecules, that synthesizes DNA using certain aspects of RNA.

reverse transcriptase inhibitor: An agent that deters or prevents RNA-directed DNA polymerase. *See also* REVERSE TRANSCRIPTASE.

Reye's syndrome: A syndrome first recognized in 1963, characterized by acute encephalopathy and fatty infiltration of the liver and possibly of the pancreas, kidney, heart, spleen, and lymph nodes.

rhinitis: Inflammation of nasal mucosa.

RIA: *See* RADIOIMMUNOASSAY.

ribavirin: A synthetic nucleoside used as an antiviral.

riboflavin: *See* VITAMIN B-2.

ribonucleic acid (RNA): A nucleic acid composed of ribonucleotide monomers. The base sequence of an RNA is dependent upon the base sequence of a section of DNA, which serves as a template for RNA synthesis (transcription). RNA controls protein synthesis in living cells, and replaces DNA in certain viruses. *See also* DEOXYRIBONUCLEIC ACID.

Rickettsia: A genus of bacteria made up of small, often multi-shaped microorganisms that are gram-negative and multiply only within the host cell. They are usually transmitted to man by fleas, lice, mites, and ticks, and are the causative agent of a variety of diseases including typhus fevers, spotted fevers, and scrub typhus.

rifabutin: A broad-spectrum antibiotic used as prophylaxis against disseminated *Mycobacterium avium* complex infection. The trade name is Mycobutin.

Rifadin: *See* RIFAMPIN.

rifampicin: *See* RIFAMPIN.

rifampin: An antibiotic synthetically derived from rifamycin that appears as a red-brown, crystalline powder. It has the antibacterial properties of the rifamycin group, and is used in the treatment of *Mycobacterium tuberculosis*. It is administered orally. Trade names are Rimactane and Rifadin. *Also called* RIFAMPICIN.

rifamycin: Any of a group of antibiotics biosynthesized by a strain of *Streptomyces mediterranei*, and effective against a broad spectrum of bacteria including gram-positive cocci, *Mycobacterium tuberculosis*, some gram-negative bacilli, and certain other mycobacteria.

right to die: The right of the patient or the patient's representative to make decisions with regard to the patient's dying such as the point at which a do not resuscitate order should be implemented.

Rimactane: *See* RIFAMPIN.

rimming: *See* ANILINGUS.

ringworm: *See* TINEA.

RIPA: *See* RADIOIMMUNOPRECIPITATION ASSAY.

risk group member: Any one of a group of individuals sharing common characteristics believed to place them at risk for infection with a communicable disease (e.g., unprotected, anal sex practitioners at risk for infection with the human immunodeficiency virus).

Ritalin: *See* METHYLPHENIDATE.

ritonavir: An HIV protease inhibitor that works by interfering with the reproductive cycle of HIV. the trade name is Norvir.

RNA: *See* RIBONUCLEIC ACID.

Robamox: *See* AMOXICILLIN.

Rolfing massage: A form of massage designed to heal body parts by strengthening the body's foundation. Rolfing involves deep massage of the tissues around muscles. The purpose is to increase the range of motion of the joints and to enhance suppleness.

route of transmission: The means by which a disease is passed or transferred from one individual to another (e.g., blood borne, exchange of body fluids, fecal to oral).

Roxicodone: *See* OXYCODONE.

Roxilox: *See* OXYCODONE.

royal jelly: A thick, milky-white creamy liquid secreted by nurse bees. It consists of vitamins A, C, D, and E, as well as being a rich source of B complex-related vitamins.

rush: *See* AMYL NITRITE INHALANT and BUTYL NITRITE INHALANT.

Ryan White CARE Act: Signed into law August 18, 1990, this legislation was designed to provide emergency assistance to localities that are disproportionately affected by the HIV epidemic. It also provides for the development and operation of essential services for individuals and families with HIV disease. CARE is an acronym for Comprehensive AIDS Resources Emergency.

Ryan White National Fund: Founded in 1986, this organization *See*ks to assist seriously ill children, particularly those with AIDS. It provides emergency financial aid, offers counseling, operates a referral service, promotes research, operates clinics, provides placement services, maintains a speakers' bureau, compiles statistics, and conducts education and awareness programs. The Fund is sponsored by Athletes and Entertainers for Kids, which is located at Nissan Motor Corporation, P.O. Box 191, Building B, Gardena, CA 90248-0191. Telephone: (213) 276-5437.

S and M: *See* SADOMASOCHISM.

sadism: (1) Obtaining sexual pleasure from dominating, hurting, or mistreating one's partner. (2) Obtaining pleasure from inflicting physical or psychological pain on another or others. (3) The opposite of masochism.

sadomasochism (S and M): (1) Obtaining sexual pleasure from the practice of sadism or masochism. (2) Obtaining pleasure from the practice of sadism or masochism.

safe sex: The practice of protecting oneself from viral transmission during sexual activities. Celibacy and masturbation are absolutely safe. The use of condoms should be employed when engaging in sexual activities that could result in the exchange of body fluids. Unprotected, casual sex should be avoided.

saliva: Fluid produced by the salivary gland and used to begin the digestive process. At one time, HIV-1 was thought to be transmitted through saliva. Some studies suggest that the proteins lysozyme and ribonuclease may neutralize the effects of HIV found in urine, tears, saliva, and breast milk.

salivary gland virus: *See* CYTOMEGALOVIRUS.

salivary-gland disease: A pathological condition involving the glands of the oral cavity that secrete saliva.

Salk vaccine: *See* POLIOVIRUS VACCINE INACTIVATED.

Salmonella: A genus of gram-negative bacteria belonging to the family Entobacteriaceae. Over 1,400 species have been identified, some of which are pathogenic. The most common manifestation is food poisoning, ranging in severity from mild gastroenteritis to death.

salmonellosis: Any disease caused by infection with bacteria of the genus *Salmonella*. It can be manifested as gastroenteritis, septicemia, or typhoid fever.

salvage therapy: Experimental or off-label treatment undertaken in patients whose illnesses have not responded to standard regimens. *See also* KITCHEN SINK THERAPY.

SAMHSA: *See* SUBSTANCE ABUSE AND MENTAL HEALTH SERVICE ADMINISTRATION.

San Francisco AIDS Foundation: Founded in 1982, this regional organization *See*ks to educate the public about AIDS prevention, and provide various social services to people with the acquired immunodeficiency syndrome. The Foundation holds education workshops, forums and seminars; disseminates educational materials and information; maintains a food bank and speakers' bureau; assists people with AIDS in obtaining emergency housing, government benefits, medical insurance, and legal referrals; conducts videotape training programs for health care providers and home health care workers to identify the needs of PWA's; produces various publications; and compiles statistics. Formerly called Kaposi's Sarcoma Research and Education Foundation. San Francisco AIDS Foundation, P.O. Box 426182, San Francisco, CA 94142-6182. Telephone: (415) 487-3000.

Sandimmune: *See* CYCLOSPORINE A.

sapphism: *See* LESBIANISM.

saquinavir: First protease inhibitor approved by the Food and Drug Administration (December 7, 1995). It was approved more quickly than any other new HIV drug at that time. Manufactured by Roche Laboratories. The trade name is Invirase.

sarsaparilla: Many different plant species are called by the general name sarsaparilla. Various species are found in Mexico, South America, and the Caribbean. True sarsaparilla, however, is obtained from tropical American species of the genus *Smilax* of the lily family. Sarsaparilla has been used for arthritis, cancer, skin diseases, and a host of other conditions. There have also been reports of its use in the treatment of psoriasis and leprosy. Sarsaparilla also has a tradition of use in various women's health concerns and has been rumored to have a progesterone-like effect. Some forms are effective as anti-venom agents and are used widely in parts of the world where snakebites are common.

scabies: A highly contagious dermatitis (skin inflammation) caused by *Sarcoptes scabies*, the itch mite. It is transmitted by close contact, and is characterized by the eruption of papules, vesicles, and pustules. Eczema may result from scratching. *Also called* the ITCH.

Schilling test: A diagnostic procedure that uses a radioactive form of vitamin B12 to determine whether a patient has pernicious anemia.

Schistosoma: (1) A genus of parasites or flukes, belonging to the family Schistosomatidae, class Trematoda, that thrive on blood. (2) The blood flukes.

schistosomiasis: A parasitic disease due to infestation with flukes of the genus *Schistosoma*.

SCID: *See* SEVERE COMBINED IMMUNODEFICIENCY.

scrapie disease: One of the transmissible brain diseases in which the brain degenerates to the appearance of a sponge. It is characterized by severe itching, debility, and the inability to coordinate muscle movements. Scrapie disease generally occurs in sheep and goats, and is inevitably fatal.

seborrhea: A functional disease of the sebaceous glands marked by the excessive secretion of sebum. *See also* SEBORRHEIC DERMATITIS.

seborrheic dermatitis: An acute or chronic inflammatory skin disease of unknown cause characterized by dry, moist, or greasy scaling, and yellow or brown-gray crusted patches. It tends to especially involve the scalp, but may include parts of the face, ears, genitalia, umbilicus, and supraorbital regions. *Also called* SEBORRHEA and SEBORRHEIC ECZEMA.

seborrheic eczema: *See* SEBORRHEIC DERMATITIS.

seizure: A brief disturbance in brain function that may manifest itself as loss of consciousness, loss of memory, sensory disturbance, or abnormal motor activity. It may or may not be accompanied by convulsions. Many diseases and conditions have seizures as a symptom.

selenium: A nonmetallic trace element that is an essential nutrient for a healthy diet. A deficiency in selenium has been confirmed as an independent predictor of mortality in HIV-infected children, and is associated with poor prognosis and rapid disease progression in both adults and children who are HIV infected.

self-concept: The mental image individuals hold of themselves.

self-disclosure: Major life realization, positive or negative. May refer to disease state, psychological state, or other condition.

self-identity: Understanding oneself as an individual apart from all others.

semen: A thick, opalescent, whitish secretion of the male reproductive organs released at the climax of sexual excitement. Semen is the secretory product of various organs (prostate, bulbourethral glands, seminal vesicles, and others) plus spermatozoa.

septic shock: Unchecked interruption of blood flow to vital organs because of a pathogen's spreading from its initial site to the bloodstream, overwhelming the body's natural defenses. Fatal if not successfully treated.

Septra: *See* TRIMETHOPRIM/SULFAMETHOXAZOLE.

serine: An amino acid. Interacts at the cellular level to affect the nef gene.

seroconversion: The change of a test result from negative to positive, indicating the presence of antibodies in response to infection or vaccination.

Seromycin: *See* CYCLOSERINE.

seronegative: Producing a negative result on serological tests; serologically negative; exhibiting no signs of antibody.

seropositive: Producing a positive result on serological tests; serologically positive; exhibiting definite signs of antibody.

seroprevalence: The number of individuals with evidence of antibodies against the causative agent of a disease in a given population at a specific period of time or at a particular point in time.

seroreversion: Phenomenon of an individual's testing positive for HIV antibodies, then testing negative for the antibodies, and subsequently testing positive again in the absense of risk factors for infection. Though it was a confusing occurrence in the first several years of the epidemic, improved testing methods have virtually eliminated this event.

serostatus: The state or condition of a serologic test (i.e., seronegative, seropositive).

Serostim: *See* SOMATROPIN.

sertraline: Oral antidepressant of the selective serotonin reuptake inhibitor (SSRI) class. Manufactured by Pfizer, sertraline was approved by the FDA in 1991 for the treatment of major depression, and in 1997 for the treatment of both obsessive-compulsive disorder and panic disorder. The trade name is Zoloft.

serum: (1) The clear portion of any body fluid, especially that which moistens serous membranes. (2) The clear, watery portion of the blood that separates upon clotting. (3) Blood serum from an animal that has been immunized against a pathogenic organism which is used for passive immunization.

severe combined immunodeficiency (SCID): A group of rare congenital disorders characterized by impairment of both humoral and cell-mediated immunity manifested by lack of antibody formation in response to the presence of antigens, lack of delayed hypersensitivity, and inability to reject foreign tissue transplants. Without restoration of immune function or gnotobiotic isolation, death usually occurs by the first birthday as a result of opportunistic infection.

sex club: Any of a group of facilities (usually private, for-profit) dedicated to the promotion of the pursuit of sexual pleasure, either in part or entirely (e.g., bath houses, orgy rooms).

sex education: *See* HUMAN SEXUALITY EDUCATION.

sex industry: That portion of the economy deriving profit from the promotion of sexual pleasure.

sex toy: *See* SEXUAL DEVICE.

sexual behavior: The instincts, drives, activities, and conduct associated with procreation and/or erotic pleasure.

sexual device: Any appliance designed to produce, or assist with the derivation of, sexual pleasure (e.g., dildo, vibrator).

sexual harassment: Any unsolicited, sexually motivated behavior, whether verbal or physical, that the recipient considers offensive. May occur in any setting, but only in the workplace is sexual harassment currently actionable.

sexual intercourse: The joining of the sexual organs of a male and a female human being, in which the erect penis is inserted into the vagina, and usually with the ejaculation of semen into the vagina. *See also* HOMOSEXUAL SEXUAL INTERCOURSE, ANAL INTERCOURSE, and VAGINAL INTERCOURSE.

sexual orientation: An individual's natural preference and attraction for sexual partners; a predilection for either same sex, opposite sex, or both (bisexual).

sexually transmitted disease (STD): Disease acquired as a result of sexual intercourse (heterosexual or homosexual) with an infected partner. This term is more inclusive than venereal disease, as it includes certain conditions that can also be acquired by nonsexual means (e.g., amebiasis or shigellosis).

Sézary syndrome: (1) A skin disease characterized by shedding. (2) A form of cutaneous T-cell lymphoma characterized by exfoliative dermatitis, severe itching, peripheral lymphadenopathy, and abnormal hyperchromatic mononuclear cells in the lymph nodes, skin, and peripheral blood.

shamanism: Religion found among the peoples of northern Asia and Europe. Followers of shamanism believe in an invisible world of powerful gods, demons, and spirits who are reponsive only to a religious leader called a shaman.

Shanti Project: Founded in 1975, this organization is divided into regional groups that provide volunteer counseling services to individuals and their loved ones who are affected by the acquired immunodeficiency syndrome or the human immunodeficiency virus. Volunteers are matched with clients based on a variety of identified needs in the belief that peer counseling can help the individual achieve the inner peace necessary to confront fears, frustration, isolation, and depression, and cope with sorrow and stress. It also educates health care workers and laypersons, produces various publications, organizes support groups, provides practical assistance, and offers long-term, low-cost housing to eligible people with AIDS. Shanti Project, 1546 Market Street, San Francisco, CA 94102-6007. Telephone: (415) 864-2273.

shark cartilage: Naturally occurring substance believed to cure various cancers or cause them to go into remission. No randomized clinical trial has tested the anecdotal evidence about shark cartilage's curative properties, and a community-based trial of thirteen AIDS patients with Kaposi's sarcoma showed no regression following treatment at a two- to three-month follow-up. Studies have confirmed that cartilage contains immune stimulation factors; however, a reliable, clinically sound therapy for any type of cancer using shark cartilage has not been developed.

Shiatsu massage: Developed in Japan, Shiatsu derives from traditional Chinese medicine. The word means, literally, "finger pressure" in Japanese. The objective of Shiatsu massage is to apply pressure along the longitudinal meridians of the body, through which the energy of life flows, according to traditional Chinese medicine. Pressure from the fingers and hands along these meridians is believed to have a positive influence on the flow of energy (qi in Chinese or ki in Japanese) through the body, thereby promoting health and wellness.

Shiatzu massage: *See* SHIATSU MASSAGE.

Shigella: A genus of gram-negative, nonmotile, rod-shaped bacteria of the family Enterobacteriaceae which ferment carbohydrates with acid but do not produce gas. The genus consists of several species, all of which normally inhabit the intestinal tract of humans and cause digestive disturbances ranging from diarrhea to severe dysentery.

shigellosis: The disease produced by organisms of the genus *Shigella*.

shiitake: Mushroom used in haute cuisine and also as an alternative therapy for HIV disease. In vitro studies conducted in Japan suggest some interference with HIV activity; however, no clinical evidence indicates that it is helpful in vivo against the human immunodeficiency virus.

shingles: (1) The nontechnical name for *herpes zoster*. (2) The eruption of acute, inflammatory, herpetic vesicles along the area of the affected nerve. The disease represents reactivation of varicella-zoster virus (chickenpox). *See also* HERPES ZOSTER.

shooting gallery: Any space, often abandoned or condemned buildings, occupied for the explicit use of the illegal sale and abuse of intravenous drugs.

sickle-cell anemia: (1) An inherited chronic anemia characterized by an abnormal red blood cell that contains a defective form of hemoglobin, causing the cell to become sickle-shaped when deprived of oxygen. (2) An inherited anemia characterized by the presence of crescent-shaped (sickle-shaped) erythrocytes and by accelerated hemolysis.

sickle-cell disease: *See* SICKLE-CELL ANEMIA.

side effect: The effect or action of a drug other than the one desired.

sigmoidoscope: A flexible or rigid instrument used to examine the lower colon (sigmoid flexure).

sigmoidoscopy: Inspection of the sigmoid colon (the lower portion of the descending colon, located between the iliac crest and the rectum, which is shaped like the letter S) using a sigmoidoscope.

sign: Any abnormality, discoverable upon examination of the patient, indicative of disease.

silymarin: Herbal remedy consisting of the *See*ds of the milk thistle. The British herbalist Nicholas Culpeper (1616-1654) first suggested the use of silymarin against jaundice more than 300 years ago. A study on rat livers indicated that silymarin protects against depletion of glutathione, a chronic problem in many HIV-infected persons. No clinical evidence currently indicates therapeutic value.

simian immunodeficiency virus (SIV): Any of a group of viruses structurally similar to the human immunodeficiency virus found in monkeys. *Also called* SIMIAN T-LYMPHOTROPHIC VIRUS (STLV).

simian retrovirus: Any of a group of retroviruses found in monkeys.

simian T-lymphotrophic virus (STLV): *See* SIMIAN IMMUNODEFICIENCY VIRUS.

sinusitis: Inflammation of a sinus.

SIV: *See* SIMIAN IMMUNODEFICIENCY VIRUS.

SK-Dexamethasone: *See* DEXAMETHASONE.

SK65: *See* PROPOXYPHENE.

sleep apnea: Momentary suspension of breathing during sleep. For diagnostic purposes, the suspension must last for at least 10 seconds and must occur 30 or more times in a single seven-hour period of sleep.

sleep disorder: Any of a constellation of conditions, signs, and symptoms that interfere with normal sleep.

slim disease: *See* HIV WASTING SYNDROME.

Social Security Administration: Established by Reorganization Plan No. 2 of 1946, the Administration oversees a national program of contributory social insurance whereby employees, employers, and the self-employed pay contributions that are pooled in special trust funds. For purposes of administration, the United States is divided into 10 regions, each headed by a Regional Commissioner. Each region contains a network of district offices, branch offices, and teleservice centers which serve as the contact between the Administration and the public. These installations are responsible for informing people of the purposes and provisions of programs, and their rights and responsibilities thereunder; assisting with claims filed for retirement, survivors, health, or disability insurance benefits, black lung benefits, or supplemental security income; developing and adjudicating claims; assisting certain beneficiaries in claiming reimbursement for medical expenses; conducting development of cases involving earnings records, coverage, and fraud-related questions; making rehabilitation service referrals; and assisting claimants in filing appeals on Administration determination of benefit entitlement or amount. Office of Public Inquiries, Social Security Administration, Department of Health and Human Services, 6401 Security Boulevard, Baltimore, MD 21235. Telephone: (800) 772-1213; TTY: (800) 325-0778.

social work: Professional activity in which licensed practitioners work directly to aid socioeconomically underprivileged or socially maladjusted groups or indiviuals. Medical social work is generally part of case mangement for patients in the above categories, or who have terminal illness such as HIV/AIDS or a type of cancer.

sociology: (1) Social science whose practitioners are engaged in the systematic study of all aspects of organized groups of human beings; (2) Scientific analysis of a social institution, such as prison or a church, as a functional whole and its relationship to the rest of society.

sodomy: (1) Copulation with a member of the same sex; (2) Non-coital copulation with a member of the opposite sex.

somatropin: Purified recombinant growth hormone often prescribed for HIV wasting, or cachexia. The product is administered through an injection.

sonography: *See* ULTRASONOGRAPHY.

Southern blot technique: A procedure used to separate and identify DNA sequences in which DNA fragments are separated by electrophoresis onto an agarose gel, blotted onto a nylon or nitrocellulose membrane, and hybridized with labeled nucleic acid probes.

sperm: (1) The semen or testicular secretion, containing spermatozoa, ejaculated from the male. (2) Spermatozoa.

sperm bank: Laboratory where semen is collected from donors and cryopreserved until purchases for artificial insemination. Screening of semen for HIV and other infectious and genetic diseases is currently not required by law or regulation.

spermatozoa: Plural of spermatozoon.

spermatozoon: The mature male germ cell which is formed within the seminiferous tubules of the testes. It consists of a head with a nucleus, a neck, a middle piece, and a tail, and resembles a tadpole. Spermatozoon is the element of semen concerned with reproduction, which pierces the envelope of the ovum to achieve fertilization.

spermicide: An agent that destroys spermatozoa.

spinal muscular atrophy: Progressive, degenerative disorder of motor neurons in the spinal cord, brain stem, and motor cortex, manifested by muscular weakness and wasting. One of a constellation of neurological symptoms appearing more frequently in HIV-infected patients who are living longer as a result of highly active antiretroviral therapy (HAART).

spinal puncture: *See* LUMBAR PUNCTURE.

spiramycin: An antibiotic produced from a member of the *Streptomyces* bacteria. It is administered orally.

spirulina: Type of blue-green algae used as a health food that purports to promote weight gain and to increase energy. While rich in amino acids and minerals, no anti-HIV activity has been scientifically demonstrated.

splenic fever: *See* ANTHRAX.

splenomegaly: Enlargement of the spleen.

Sporanox: *See* ITRACONAZOLE.

Sporothrix schenckii: A species of the genus *Sporothrix,* a dimorphic, imperfect fungi that is the causative agent of sporotrichosis. It grows in soil or vegetation (especially in thorny bushes), and is transmitted when infected thorns enter subcutaneous tissues. It also grows as a yeast, and parasitizes tissue as a yeast at 37°C.

sporotrichosis: A chronic fungal infection caused by *Sporothrix schenckii* that is characterized by abscesses, nodules, and ulcers of the skin and adjacent lymph nodes. The infection may remain localized, or it may spread throughout the body via the bloodstream.

sprue: A disease characterized by weakness, weight loss, anemia, and malabsorption of essential elements. It occurs in both tropical and nontropical forms, and the cause is unknown.

sputum: Matter ejected from the bronchi, lungs, and trachea through the mouth.

sputum examination: The microscopic inspection of expectorated matter (especially mucus or mucopurulent matter ejected in diseases involving the air passages) for the purpose of diagnosis.

SPV-30: Herbal compound synthesized from the evergreen boxwood. Some buyers' clubs sold the compound, touting its alleged anti-HIV properties. Such activity has yet to be scientifically demonstrated.

squamous cell: A flat, scalelike, epithelial cell.

squamous cell carcinoma: A malignant tumor developing from squamous epithelium.

St. Johns wort: *See* HYPERICIN.

Staphylococcus: A genus of aerobic to facultatively anaerobic, nonmotile, nonspore-forming bacteria containing gram-positive, spherical cells that divide in multiple planes to form irregular clusters resembling grapes. Under anaerobic conditions, they produce lactic acid from glucose; under aerobic conditions, they produce acetic acid and small amounts of carbon dioxide. Certain strains (coagulase-positive) produce various toxins that are potentially pathogenic, and may cause food poisoning. They are found on the skin, skin glands, mucous and nasal membranes, and in various food products.

Staphylococcus aureus: A species of *Staphylococcus* commonly found on the skin and mucous membranes, especially those of the mouth and nose. They are characterized by the production of golden-yellow pigment, and are gram-positive and coagulase positive. They cause serious suppurative conditions and systemic diseases. Various strains of the species produce toxins that cause food poisoning and toxic shock syndrome.

stavudine (d4T): Fourth drug approved by the Food and Drug Administration for treatment of HIV/AIDS on June 27, 1994. It joined three other nucleoside analogs: zidovudine, didanosine, and zalcitabine. Stavudine was the first drug granted parallel track status by the FDA. It was approved a regulatory mechanism known as accelerated approval. The trade name is Zerit, and it is manufactured by Bristol-Myers Squibb. Early in its development it was known as d4T.

STD: *See* SEXUALLY TRANSMITTED DISEASE.

sterilization: (1) The destruction of all microorganisms in, on, or about an object by employing various means such as chemical agents (alcohol, ethylene oxide gas, phenol), high-velocity electron bombardment, steam, or ultraviolet light radiation. (2) The act or process by which an individual is made incapable of reproduction or fertilization (e.g., castration, tubectomy, vasectomy).

Stevens-Johnson syndrome: A form of erythema multiforme (eruption of dark red papules or tubercles) that is sometimes fatal. It is characterized by systemic exfoliative mucocutaneous lesions, some of which may be severe. The lesions may involve the ears, nose, lips, eyes, anus, genitals, lungs, gastrointestinal tract, heart, and kidneys.

stigma: (1) A mark of disgrace or reproach. (2) Something that detracts from the character of a person or group.

STLV: *See* SIMIAN VIRUS T-LYMPHOTROPHIC.

stomatitis: Inflammation of the mouth.

straight: *See* HETEROSEXUAL.

streptomycin: A bacterial antibiotic derived from the soil microbe, *Streptomyces griseus*. It belongs to the aminoglycoside class, and is effective against most gram-negative and acid-fast bacteria. It is also effective against certain gram-positive forms, but it is used mainly in the treatment of tuberculosis.

stroke: A condition characterized by paralysis and often some irreversible neurologic damage. It can include focal weakness, speech impediment, with impaired consciousness; it is caused by acute vascular lesions of the brain such as hemorrhage, embolism, or thrombosis. *Also called* CEREBROVASCULAR ACCIDENT and STROKE SYNDROME.

stroke syndrome: *See* STROKE.

Strongyloides stercoralis: A roundworm occurring in tropical or subtropical countries, or in the southern United States that infects dogs, primates, and humans. The female and larvae inhabit the intestines of the host, where they cause diarrhea and ulceration. The rod-shaped larvae are expelled in the stool, and may pass through the venous system to the lungs where they cause hemorrhage (pulmonary strongyloidiasis). From the lungs they migrate upward, and reach the intestines via the trachea and esophagus. Infestation may persist for years due to the nature of the life cycle. Massive infections may be seen in patients treated with immunosuppressive drugs or in immunosuppressed patients. Infection may be fatal.

strongyloidiasis: Infection with nematodes of the genus *Strongyloides*. Infection can occur indirectly by larvae of a new generation developed in the soil; directly by infective larvae developed without an intervening adult phase; or by autoreinfection where larvae develop within the intestinal feces of the host, penetrate the mucosa, and migrate back to the intestines through blood-lung interactions. Autoreinfection is the cause of most serious human infections and the majority of fatalities. *Also called* STRONGYLOIDOSIS. *See also* STRON-GYLOIDES STERCORALIS.

strongyloidosis: *See* STRONGYLOIDIASIS.

subacute encephalitis: *See* AIDS DEMENTIA COMPLEX.

substance abuse: Use or overuse of any substance (e.g., caffeine, nicotine, alcohol, pharmaceuticals, designer drugs) that produces negative health effects. *See also* DRUG ABUSE.

Substance Abuse and Mental Health Service Administation (SAMHSA): Part of the Department of Health and Human Services, Public Health Service, SAMHSA was established in 1992 as a successor to the Alcohol, Drug Abuse, and Mental Health Administration, which dated from 1974. SAMHSA coordinates federal programs, and works to improve the quality and availability of substance abuse treatment, and prevention and mental health services. They accomplish their work through three centers: the Center for Mental Health Services, the Center for Substance Abuse Prevention, and the Center for Substance Abuse Treatment. Substance Abuse and Mental Health Service Administration, 5600 Fishers Lane, Rockville, MD 20857. Telephone: (301) 443-8956. Spanish language materials are available directly from the Web site, <http://www.samhsa.gov/>.

suicide: The termination of one's own life.

sulfadiazine: A derivative of sulfonamide that appears as a white or yellowish powder. Because of its ability to penetrate the blood-brain barrier, it is used in the treatment of some types of meningitis. Sulfadiazine is also used to treat infections involving susceptible organisms such as acute urinary tract infections and chancroid. It is administered orally.

sulfamethoxazole: A sulfonamide appearing as a white to off-white crystalline powder that is used in the treatment of urinary tract infections. It is administered orally.

sulfonamide: Any of a group of compounds that consist of the amides of sulfamic acid. They are derivatives of sulfanilamide, and are bacteriostatic. Their action on bacteria results from their ability to interfere with the functioning of the enzyme systems required for normal metabolism, growth, and multiplication.

Supplementary Security Income (SSI): A basic Federal payment program administered by the Social Security Administration for the aged, blind, and disabled. It is financed out of general revenue. *See also* SOCIAL SECURITY ADMINISTRATION.

support group: A group of individuals whose purpose is to mutually give courage, confidence, or faith. Most often associated with psychotherapy. *See also* SUPPORT NETWORK.

support network: A group of interconnected or cooperative individuals who give courage, confidence, or faith to each other. A support network tends to be less formal in nature than a support group (e.g., family or friends).

suppressor cell: A subset of T lymphocytes that inhibits B lymphocyte antibody formation, and is involved in autoimmunity and immune tolerance. *See also* LYMPHOCYTE.

suppurative: Forming pus.

suramin: The first compound identified in 1984 with anti-HIV activity in vitro, it entered clinical trials for patients with Kaposi's sarcoma and AIDS-related complex. The drug was found to be highly toxic, with no clinical, immunologic, or virologic benefit to HIV-infected individuals.

surgeon general: The chief medical officer in the U.S. Army, Air Force, Navy, and Public Health Service.

surgery: Type of therapy that uses operative procedures to cure or diagnose some diseases, to repair or correct deformities, and to repair injuries. Also the branch of medicine concerned with these procedures.

surveillance: (1) The monitoring, watching, or controlling of something. (2) The procedure of closely monitoring the contacts of individuals exposed to an infectious disease during the incubation period to prevent the spread of the disease. Surveillance is used in place of quarantine. *See also* QUARANTINE.

susceptible host: Any organism that is easily invaded by a parasitic organism for the purpose of subsistence, especially for nourishment.

Sustiva: *See* EFAVIRENZ.

sweat: *See* PERSPIRATION.

Swedish massage: System of massage that first became popular in the West. The Swede Pir Henrik Ling (1776-1839) used what was known of physiology in the nineteenth century to develop a therapeutic modality that combined massage with physical exercise. Both the therapy and the terminology he used are still practiced today.

symptom: (1) Any perceptive change in the body or bodily functions indicative of disease, kinds of disease, or phases of disease. They may be classed as objective, subjective, cardinal, and constitutional. Generally though, all symptoms are classed as subjective, with objective indications being considered signs. (2) Any change in a patient's condition indicative of mental or physical illness.

syncope: A transient loss of consciousness due to inadquate blood flow to the brain.

synergy: Action of two or more agents or drugs working together; cooperation.

syphilis: A subacute to chronic, infectious, venereal disease characterized by lesions that may involve any organ or body tissue. Generally, cutaneous manifestations are exhibited, and relapses may occur frequently. Syphilis may remain asymptomatic for years. It is usually transmitted through sexual contact (both heterosexual and homosexual), but it may be acquired in utero or by direct contact with infected tissue or blood. If untreated, syphilis progresses through three clinical stages: primary (initial painless ulceration lesions—chancre—at the site of inoculation), secondary (widespread mucocutaneous lesions and generalized regional lymphadenopathy), and tertiary (destructive lesions involving many organs and tissues, including the heart and central nervous system).

systemic: (1) Relating to the entire organism as distinguished from any of its individual parts. (2) Relating to a system.

systemic disease: Any pathologic condition involving the entire organism as opposed to an individual organ system or part.

T

T cell: *See* T LYMPHOCYTE.

T lymphocyte: A thymocyte-derived lymphocyte that is long-lived, and of immunological importance since it is responsible for cell-mediated immunity. *Also called* T CELL.

T lymphocyte, helper cell: CD4 lymphocyte. *See also* HELPER CELL and LYMPHOCYTE.

T lymphocyte, suppressor cell: CD8 lymphocyte. *See also* SUPPRESSOR CELL and LYMPHOCYTE.

tai chi: Ancient system of sets of slow movements derived originally from the martial arts and sometimes described as "meditation for the body." The objective is to promote the circulation of qi, or life-giving force, within the body, thereby enhancing health and well-being.

tat gene: The gene which encodes a transactivating genetic element of the human immunodeficiency virus that increases the production of cellular and viral proteins.

tattoo: Form of body marking that makes a generally indelible mark or figure on the body by the insertion of pigment under the skin, usually with needles. HIV, hepatitis B, and hepatitis C can all be transmitted through this procedure if sterile instruments are not used.

taurine: Nutrient essential during mammalian development and present in bile. It is a derivative of cysteine.

Taxol: *See* PACLITAXEL.

T-cell count: Calculation of the number of T lymphocytes in a cubic millimeter of blood.

T-cell leukemia: *See* T-CELL LYMPHOMA.

T-cell lymphoma: An acute or subacute disease associated with a human T cell virus, and characterized by lymphadenopathy, hypercalcemia, hepatosplenomegaly, skin lesions, and peripheral blood involvement. *Also called* T-CELL LEUKEMIA.

T-cell ratio: The ratio of T4 lymphocytes (helper cells) to T8 lymphocytes (suppressor cells) in the blood.

tears: Watery, saline solution continuously produced by the lacrimal glands in the eye. Tears serve both to lubricate the eyes and to help dispose of irritants that may sometimes enter the eyes. Although HIV may be present in the tears of an infected individual, the amount is so small that it the virus cannot be transmitted through contact with these tears.

Teens Teaching AIDS Prevention: Founded in 1987, this organization seeks to inform teenagers about HIV and AIDS through peer education. It operates a toll-free hotline staffed by trained teenagers with adult advisers, maintains a speakers' bureau, and provides companions for youths with AIDS. Teens Teaching AIDS Prevention, 3030 Walnut, Kansas City, MO 64108. Telephone: (816) 561-8784 or toll-free (800) 234-TEEN (hotline).

telephone triage: Use of a trained operator to determine the gravity of a sick person's complaint.

terminal stage: Pertaining to the end phase.

testicular atrophy: A wasting away, or decrease in size and function, of the testis (male reproductive gland located in the cavity of the scrotum).

testicular cancer: *See* TESTICULAR CARCINOMA.

testicular carcinoma: A malignant neoplasm occurring in the male reproductive gland (testis).

testing: (1) The procedure used to determine the presence or nature of a substance or disease. (2) Producing a significant chemical reaction.

tetracycline: Any of a group of broad-spectrum antibiotics belonging to certain species of *Streptomyces*. They may also be produced semisynthetically. The tetracyclines are effective against a variety of organisms, including gram-negative and gram-positive bacteria, chlamydias, mycoplasmas, rickettsias, and some viruses and protozoa. Trade names are Tetracyn and SK-Tetracycline.

Tetracyn: *See* TETRACYCLINE.

T4 cells: Helper cells which assist in the production of antibody-forming cells from B lymphocytes. *See also* T LYMPHOCYTE.

thalidomide: Notorious for causing severe birth defects among children whose mothers took this drug during pregnancy, thalidomide has recently been shown to be an excellent therapy for several serious disorders, including HIV wasting or cachexia and AIDS-associated diarrhea. The drug currently has orphan drug status from the Food and Drug Administration for these disorders.

theosophy: Originating in the United States in 1875, theosophy borrows heavily from Buddhist teachings, particularly regarding reincarnation. More broadly, theosophy refers to any teaching about or conceptualization of a supreme being based on mystical insight.

therapeutic touch: Grounded in nursing research, practitioners of therapeutic touch promote relaxation, reduction of pain, and relief of anxiety by focusing energy through the hands to facilitate healing. Developed in the early 1970s by a registered nurse and a natural healer, the therapy remains controversial.

therapy: The treatment of a disease or pathological condition. *See also* TREATMENT.

thiamin: B vitamin whose deficiency causes beriberi. Thiamine is water soluble.

thiethylperazine: A dopamine antagonist that is particularly useful in treating the nausea and vomiting associated with anesthesia, mildly emetic cancer chemotherapy agents, radiation therapy, and toxins. Trade name is Torecan.

thistle: *See* SILYMARIN.

3TC: *See* LAMIVUDINE.

threonine: An essential amino acid.

thrombocytopenia: A condition in which there is a decrease in the number of platelets in circulating blood. *Also called* THROMBOPENIA.

thrombopenia: *See* THROMBOCYTOPENIA.

thrush: *See* ORAL CANDIDIASIS.

thymidine: (1) A nucleoside that is one of the basic components of deoxyribonucleic acid. (2) A nucleoside present in deoxyribonucleotide.

TIA: *See* TRANSIENT ISCHEMIC ATTACK.

Tinactin: *See* TOLNAFTATE.

tinea: Any fungus skin disease involving various parts of the body, with the specific type indicating the part involved (e.g., tinea barbae [beard]). *Also called* RINGWORM.

tinea pedis: Fungal skin disease that occurs on the foot; commonly called athlete's foot.

tissue bank: Any facility that collects, processes, and stores tissue for subsequent transplantation. Tissues are tested for various pathogens and are stored in either a freeze-dried or frozen state. *See also* BLOOD BANK.

TMP/SMX: *See* TRIMETHOPRIM/SULFAMETHOXAZOLE.

Tofranil: *See* IMIPRAMINE.

tolnaftate: A synthetic antifungal agent appearing as a white to creamy white powder. It is used topically in treating various forms of tinea. The trade name is Tinactin.

toot: *See* COCAINE.

topical: Pertaining to a specific surface area on the body.

Torecan: *See* THIETHYLPERAZINE.

torulosis: *See* CRYPTOCOCCOSIS.

total parenteral nutrition (TPN): Provision of all of an adult's nutritional needs intravenously, either through a central line (long-term) or peripheral total parenteral nutrition, if the patient needs nutritional support for 10 or fewer days.

toxic shock syndrome (TSS): A rare disease caused by toxins that are produced by certain strains of *Staphylococcus aureus* bacteria. It is characterized by acute high fever, diarrhea, vomiting, and myalgia (tenderness or pain in the muscles), followed by hypotension and possible death due to shock. It mostly affects young menstruating women using tampons, but cases have been diagnosed in nonmenstruating women, young boys, and men.

toxicity: The quality of being poisonous.

Toxoplasma gondii: An intracellular, nonhost-specific, widespread, sporozoan species that is parasitic in a variety of vertebrates including humans. The sexual cycle, leading to the production of oocysts, develops exclusively in cats and other felines. Infection from ingestion of oocysts, tissue cysts in raw meat, or transplacental migration allows the proliferative stages and tissue cysts to develop in a variety of animal species in utero. It is the causative agent of toxoplasmosis.

toxoplasmosis: An acute or chronic disease caused by infection with the protozoa *Toxoplasma gondii*. The organism is found in many mammals and birds, but the definitive host is the feces of cats. In humans, infection is usually asymptomatic. When symptoms do appear, they may range from a mild, self-limited disease similar to mononucleosis to a more severe, disseminated disease (encephalitis, hepatitis, or pneumonitis) causing extensive damage to the brain, central nervous system, liver, and lungs. The immunocompromised patient and transplacentally infected fetus are the most susceptible to severe manifestations.

TPN: *See* TOTAL PARENTERAL NUTRITION.

trace minerals: Organic elements found in minute quantities in foods and human tissues but that are nonetheless essential for good health. Examples are zinc and iron.

Trade-Related Aspects of Intellectual Property Rights Agreement (TRIPS): Most comprehensive multilateral agreement on intellectual property currently in existence internationally. Disputes among members are settled through the World Trade Organisation. The agreement covers patents and is currently contentious in the AIDS arena because of the pressing need for prohibitively expensive, life-saving anti-HIV drugs in sub-Saharan Africa. Manufacturers there want to produce generic forms of some drugs, in violation of the patent rights of multinational pharmaceutical companies.

traditional healer: Person in African traditional medicine who typically treats disease by relying on herbs, animal spirits, and spiritual counseling rather than emphasizing the cause of disease and attempting to treat the pathogen.

transference: Psychological process in which a patient shifts patterns of behavior, thought, and feeling from an authority figure (such as a parent) to a caregiver or health professional.

transfusion: The injection of whole blood or a blood component into the bloodstream.

transfusion-associated AIDS: The development of the acquired immunodeficiency syndrome as a result of a transfusion with HIV-infected blood or blood components.

transgenderist: An individual who adopts both masculine and feminine attitudes, behaviors, and characteristics.

transient ischemic attack (TIA): The temporary interruption of the blood supply to the brain. The symptoms and signs of neurologic deficit may last from a few minutes to hours but are not persistent. No evidence of residual brain damage or neurologic damage exists after the attack.

transmission: (1) The conveyance of disease from one individual to another. (2) The passage of a nerve impulse across an anatomic cleft by activating a special chemical mediator, which stimulates the structure across the synapse. (3) Transfer.

transplantation: Movement of tissue or an organ from one person to another (e.g., kidney transplantation) or from one part of person's body to another (e.g., skin graft at the site of a burn).

transsexual: (1) An individual who has had his/her external anatomy surgically changed to that of the opposite sex. (2) An individual who practices transsexualism.

transsexualism: (1) The desire to surgically change one's anatomic sexual characteristics to conform with that of the opposite sex. (2) The state of being a transsexual.

transvestism: The practice of dressing in the clothes of the opposite sex, especially the adoption of feminine clothing and characteristics by a male.

transvestite: An individual who exhibits transvestism.

trazodone: A drug used in the treatment of any type of depression. It is also used to reduce the symptoms of agoraphobia, drug induced insomnia, essential tremor, repetitive screaming, and some pain syndromes. Trade name is Desyrel.

treatment: Medical, pharmaceutical, or surgical management of a patient.

treatment protocol: Written plan for the steps to be followed in an experiment.

treatment-experienced: Patients with a history of having been treated for a specific condition with a particular drug. HIV monotherapy has been shown to promote the growth of treatment-resistant virus, so many treatment-experienced HIV patients are unable to get their viral load to undetectable levels. *See also* TREATMENT-NAÏVE.

treatment-naïve: Patients with no history of having been treated for a specific condition with a particular drug. HIV patients who have not been subjected to monotherapy have the best chance of driving their viral load to undetectable levels with a combination therapy. *See also* TREATMENT-EXPERIENCED.

Treponema pallidum: The causative agent of syphilis in humans.

triage: The sorting out and classifying of sick, injured, or wounded persons. This term was developed during wartime, and is used in times of disaster. Triage determines the priority of medical need of patients; it assigns placement for treatment in order of severity, life threatening nature, and survival potential. It provides a way to promote efficient use of health care personnel, facilities, and equipment to the maximum benefit of all patients.

trial accrual: The number of persons enrolled in a clinical trial at a given time.

Trichomonas hominis: *See* PENTATRICHOMONAS HOMINIS.

Trichomonas vaginalis: A species of parasitic protozoan flagellates, belonging to the genus *Trichomonas,* that are commonly found in the urethra and vagina of women and in the urethra and prostate gland of men. It is the causative agent of trichomoniasis vaginitis.

trichomoniasis vaginitis: Acute or subacute urethritis or vaginitis due to infection with *Trichomonas vaginalis* that does not invade the tissue or mucosa but causes an inflammatory reaction. Infection is venereal or by other forms of contact; usually asymptomatic but may produce vaginitis, with vulvar and vaginal pruritus, vaginal discharge of white or yellowish viscid fluid containing mucus and pus, and rarely purulent urethritis in males.

trimethoprim: An antimicrobial agent that enhances the effect of sulfonamides and sulfones.

trimethoprim/sulfamethoxazole (TMP/SMX): A drug combination of trimethoprim and sulfamethoxazole that is used in the treatment of *Pneumocystis carinii* pneumonia and infection with *Isospora belli*. Trade names are Bactrim and Septra.

trimetrexate: An antineoplastic agent and antiprotozoal orphan drug used in the treatment of *Pneumocystis carinii* pneumonia. The trade name is Neutrexin.

Trimox: *See* AMOXICILLIN.

trip: A vernacular term used to denote a drug-induced period of hallucination or euphoria.

TRIPS: *See* TRADE-RELATED ASPECTS OF INTELLECTUAL PROPERTY RIGHTS AGREEMENT.

trust: Essential ingredient of the health care provider-patient relationship. The provider trusts the patient to be compliant with instructions, and the patient trusts the provider to provide the most efficacious therapy possible for a given condition.

tryptophan: An essential amino acid, necessary for normal growth and development.

TSS: *See* TOXIC SHOCK SYNDROME.

tubercle: (1) A granulomatous lesion caused by infection with *Mycobacterium tuberculosis*. They vary in size and in histologic component proportions; but tend to be circumscribed, firm, spheroidal lesions that generally consist of three zones: (a) an inner focus of necrosis, (b) a middle zone consisting of an accumulation of large mononuclear phagocytes (macrophages): Langhans type multinucleated giant cells may also be present, and (c) an outer zone consisting mostly of numerous lymphocytes with a few monocytes and plasma cells. Where healing has begun, fibrous tissue forming at the periphery may form a fourth zone. (2) A term used nonspecifically to refer to granuloma.

tuberculosis: Any infectious disease caused by the *Mycobacterium,* with the most common causative agent being *Mycobacterium tuberculosis.* It is characterized by inflammatory infiltrations, formation of tubercles, caseous necrosis, abscesses, calcification, and fibrosis. Tuberculosis most commonly affects the respiratory system, but it may affect other parts of the body such as the gastrointestinal tract, bones, and skin. Infection is usually through contact with an infected person or animal.

Tylox: *See* OXYCODONE.

typhoid fever: (1) An acute infectious disease, acquired by ingesting food or water contaminated by waste matter excreted from the body, characterized by fever. (2) An acute infectious disease characterized by sustained bacteremia and infestation of the pathogen within the mononuclear phagocytic cells of the liver, lymph nodes, spleen, and Peyer's patches of the ileum, accompanied by fever, rash, headache, malaise, and abdominal pain. Diagnosis is made by isolation of the bacteria from the blood.

typhus: An acute infectious disease caused by *rickettsiae,* and occurring in two forms: endemic typhus (murine) and epidemic typhus (louse-borne).

tyrosine: An essential amino acid present in many proteins.

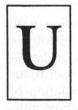

ulcer: A local defect, lesion, or open sore of the skin or mucous membrane that is accompanied by the sloughing of inflammatory necrotic (dead or decaying) tissue. Pus may be discharged if the sore becomes infected.

ulceration: (1) The development or formation of an ulcer. (2) An ulcer.

ultrasonic cardiography: *See* ECHOCARDIOGRAPHY.

ultrasonography: The use of ultrasonic waves to visualize or photograph an organ or tissue by recording the echoes or pulses of the waves as they are projected from the tissues.

UNAIDS: *See* JOINT UNITED NATIONS PROGRAM ON AIDS.

United Nations: United Nations Headquarters GA-57, New York, NY 10017. Telephone: (212) 963-4475.

universal precautions: Guidelines whose purpose is to protect workers who risk exposure to blood-borne pathogens in the workplace. First proposed by the Centers for Disease Control in 1985, they were mandated by the Occupational Safety and Health Administration for all U.S. workers in health care settings in 1991.

unprotected sexual behavior: Sexual contact without the benefit of any type of barrier protection against unwanted pregnancy or sexually transmitted diseases.

uremia: (1) An excessive amount of nitrogenous substances (e.g., urea or creatinine) in the blood that is normally excreted by the kidney. (2) The constellation of symptoms associated with the toxic condition caused by chronic or acute renal failure including anorexia, nausea, and vomiting. *See also* AZOTEMIA.

urethritis: Inflammation of the urethra.

urine: Waste fluid excreted by the kidneys through the urethra.

urolagnia: Sexual stimulation associated with the sight of a person urinating. *See also* WATER SPORT and GOLDEN SHOWER.

urology: Study of the urinary system in both males and females and of the genital tract in males. Also, the branch of medicine concerned with the same.

U.S. Commission on Civil Rights (USCCR): The USCCR was first established by Congress in 1957 as an independent, bipartisan agency. The commission investigates complaints regarding disenfranchisement and denial of equal protection of the laws because of race, color, religion, sex, disability, or national origin. U.S. Commission on Civil Rights, 624 9th Street N.W., Washington, DC 20425. Telephone: (202) 376-8312. E-mail is available directly from the Web site, <http://www.usccr.gov/>.

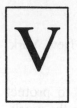

VA: *See* DEPARTMENT OF VETERANS' AFFAIRS.

vaccination: The introduction of any vaccine into the body to establish resistance to a specific infectious disease. *See also* IMMUNIZATION.

vaccine: The incorporation of weakened or killed microorganisms with a suitable liquid for administration in order to prevent or treat an infectious disease.

vacuolar myelopathy: A pathologic condition involving vacuolization (the formation of vacuoles) and sometimes degeneration of the spinal cord.

vacuole: (1) A clear place in the substance of a cell. Sometimes it is degenerative in character; sometimes it surrounds a foreign body and serves as a temporary stomach for digestion of that foreign matter. (2) A minute space found in any tissue.

vaginal digital intercourse: Insertion of a finger or fingers into the vagina for the purpose of obtaining sexual pleasure.

vaginal intercourse: Sexual intercourse by insertion of the penis into the vagina.

vaginal manual intercourse: Insertion of the hand into the vagina for the purpose of obtaining sexual pleasure.

vaginal secretion: (1) The substance produced by glands in the vagina. (2) The process whereby cells of the glands in the vagina produce materials from the blood.

vaginitis: Inflammation of the vagina.

valine: Essential amino acid derived from the digestion of proteins. Normal infant growth is dependent on this amino acid.

Valium: *See* DIAZEPAM.

valley fever: *See* COCCIDIOIDOMYCOSIS.

varicella-zoster virus: A herpetovirus, structurally identical to herpes simplex virus, that causes herpes zoster and varicella (chickenpox) in humans. Herpes zoster results from secondary infection by varicella-zoster virus or by reactivation of infection, which may have been latent for some years; varicella results from primary infection with varicella-zoster virus.

vasopressin: (1) A hormone formed by the neuronal cells of the hypothalamic nuclei, and transported to the posterior lobe of the hypophysis (pituitary gland) where it is stored through the hypothalamo-hypophyseal tract. It stimulates the contraction of the muscular tissue of the capillaries and arterioles, elevating blood pressure. (2) A pharmaceutical preparation of similar nature, extracted from the posterior pituitary of domestic animals or produced synthetically. It is used as an antidiuretic in the treatment of acute or chronic diabetes insipidus. Also called antidiuretic hormone. The trade name is Pitressin.

VD: *See* VENEREAL DISEASE.

venereal disease (VD): Any pathologic condition acquired through sexual intercourse (heterosexual or homosexual) with an infected partner. *See also* SEXUALLY TRANSMITTED DISEASE.

venereal wart: *See* CONDYLOMA ACUMINATUM.

vertical transmission: *See* PERINATAL TRANSMISSION.

Veterans Benefits Administration: The Administration conducts an integrated program of veterans benefits including compensation and pension, vocational rehabilitation and education, loan guaranty, and veterans assistance. It is one of three organizations which constitute the Department of Veterans Affairs, and has a central office as well as field facilities. Public Affairs Officer, Veterans Benefits Administration, Department of Veterans Affairs, 1800 G. Street N.W., Room 520, Washington, DC 20223. Telephone: (202) 273-6761.

Veterans' Employment and Training Service (VETS): Operating as part of the Department of Labor, VETS coordinates employment information and training programs for veterans of the armed forces. U.S. Department of Labor, VETS Office of Public Affairs, 200 Constitution Avenue, N.W., Room S-1310A, Washington, DC 20210. Telephone: (202) 219-5573; Web site, <http://www.dol.gov/dol/vets/>.

viatical: Financial settlement in which a person suffering from a terminal illness sells or transfers ownership of a life insurance policy to a person or a company, getting a percentage of the face value of the policy in exchange. Before the development of antiviral drugs that increased life span for some HIV-infected persons, viatical settlements were very popular because they provided cash for medical care, travel, or other needs or desires of the patient.

vidarabine: An antiviral agent that inhibits DNA synthesis, and is effective in the treatment of herpes simplex and herpes zoster-varicella viruses. It has also been show to be effective against herpes simplex encephalitis. *Also called* ADENINE ARABINOSIDE and ARA-A. The trade name is Vira-A.

Videx: *See* DIDANOSINE.

vif gene: The gene in the human immunodeficiency virus that encodes proteins of 23,000 molecular weight and affects virus replication by increasing virus production.

villoma: *See* PAPILLOMA.

villous papilloma: *See* PAPILLOMA.

villous tumor: *See* PAPILLOMA.

vinblastine sulfate: (1) A drug that prevents the development, growth, or proliferation of malignant cells. (2) An antineoplastic drug obtained from *Vinca rosea* used in the treatment of Hodgkin's disease, Kaposi's sarcoma, choriocarcinoma, acute and chronic leukemias, and other neoplastic disorders. *See also* VINCRISTINE SULFATE.

vincristine sulfate: (1) A drug that prevents the development, growth, or proliferation of malignant cells. (2) An antineoplastic drug obtained from *Vinca rosea* with similar activity to vinblastine, but is more useful in the treatment of acute leukemia and lymphocytic lymphosarcoma.

Vira-A: *See* VIDARABINE.

Viracept: *See* NELFINAVIR.

viral breakthrough: Detection of HIV in a person who, through the use of potent drug cocktails, had driven the virus to undetectable levels in the bloodstream.

viral encephalitis: Encephalitis caused by a virus.

viral load: Amount of human immunodeficiency virus RNA per milliliter of blood plasma, as measured by polymerase chain reaction and bDNA tests. Viral load indicates both virus concentration and reproduction rate. The measurement of viral load has largely replaced T-cell count as a predictor of disease progression.

Viramune: *See* NEVIRAPINE.

virology: The study of viruses and viral diseases.

virus: A minute infectious organism not visible under an ordinary light microscope. These organisms are, however, visible in electron microscopy. It is characterized by its entire dependency upon host cells for its metabolic and reproductive needs. Viruses consist of nucleic acid, a strand of DNA or RNA (but not both), and a protein covering. Viruses may be classified according to the host they dominate: bacteria, animal, or plant. They are also classed according to their origin, mode of transmission, manifestation they produce in the host, and geographic location where they are first isolated.

Visiting Nurse Associations of America: Founded in 1983, this organization consists of voluntary, nonprofit, home health care agencies. It *See*ks to develop competitive strength among its members, develop business resources, institute economic programs, issue public service announcements, produce various publications, and conduct workshops and training seminars. Visiting Nurse Associations of America, c/o Pam Hamilton, 3801 E. Florida, Suite 900, Denver, CO 80210. Telephone: (303) 753-0218.

visna: A viral disease that affects sheep. The primary target is the central nervous system. It is characterized by asymptomatic onset and partial paralysis of the hind limbs, progressing to total paralysis and death.

Vistaril Parenteral: *See* HYDROXYZINE.

Vistide: *See* CIDOFOVIR.

visualization: Relaxation and stress reduction technique that involves imagining particular events, scenes, or outcomes. *See also* GUIDED IMAGERY.

vitamin A: Fat-soluble vitamin formed in the body from leafy green and yellow vegetables, butter, liver, and egg yolks. When taken as a supplement, Vitamin A is toxic in large doses.

vitamin B-1: Part of the B-complex of vitamins, Vitamin B-1 is also known as thiamine. Whole grains, legumes, nuts, and egg yolks are all good sources for this nutrient.

vitamin B-2: Part of the B-complex of vitamins, Vitamin B-2 is water-soluble and is also known as riboflavin. All meats, legumes, egg yolks, and nuts are good sources for this nutrient.

vitamin B-6: Part of the B-complex of vitamins, Vitamin B-6 is also known as pyridoxine. Good sources for this nutrient, essential for the metabolism of amino acids, are meats, grains, and nuts.

vitamin B-12: Substance extracted from the liver that is essential for the production of red blood cells. It is used therapeutically for diseases in which formation of red blood cells is defective.

vitamin C: Also known as ascorbic acid, Vitamin C is essential for healthy tissues and for the formation of collagen in connective tissue. Some have speculated that it can prevent the common cold, or at least decrease the severity of symptoms.

vitamin D: Fat soluble vitamin essential for normal development of bones and teeth. Present in milk products, fish oils, and egg yolks.

vitamin deficiency: Insufficient quantity of a vitamin in the body. Such deficiency can lead to diseases such as scurvy (Vitamin C deficiency), can slow normal growth and development, or can lead to general malaise.

vitamin E: Powerful antioxidant that is an essential nutrient for human beings. *Also known as* ALPHA-TOCOPHEROL.

vitamin K: Fat soluble vitamin that is essential for blood to clot; its absence or deficiency leads to hemorrhage.

vitamin M: *See* FOLIC ACID.

vitamin therapy: Use of a vitamin to treat a disease or condition.

Vitravene: *See* FOMIVIRSEN.

voluntary testing: Agreeing to be tested for HIV of one's own volition, rather than secretly or by mandate.

von Willebrand's disease: A congenital bleeding disorder. It usually manifests at an early age, with the symptoms decreasing with age or during pregnancy. It is characterized by prolonged periods of bleeding, deficient amount of coagulation factor VIII in the blood, and is associated with increased bleeding during surgery or trauma, and excessive loss of blood during menstruation.

vpr gene: A gene in the human immunodeficiency virus whose function is presently unknown.

vulvovaginal condition: The state of health pertaining to the vulva and vagina.

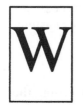 **Warren Grant Magnuson Clinical Center:** One of the centers of the National Institutes of Health (NIH), the Magnuson Clinical Center is the clinical research center of the NIH and provides the patient care, services, and environment necessary to conduct clinical trials and training on the NIH campus. Warren Grant Magnuson Clinical Center, National Institutes of Health, Bethesda, MD 20892. Telephone: (800) 411-1222; Fax: (301) 480-9793. E-mail is available directly from the Web site, <http://www.cc.nih.gov/>.

wart: A circumscribed elevation of the skin resulting from an increase in size or bulk of the epidermis and the protuberances in the layer just under the epidermis. Warts are caused by a *papillomavirus*.

wasting syndrome: *See* HIV WASTING SYNDROME.

water sport: Sexual activity involving urination. This may include watching others urinate or having someone urinate on their body. *See also* UROLAGNIA and GOLDEN SHOWER.

Watkins Commission: *See* PRESIDENTIAL COMMISSION ON THE HUMAN IMMUNODEFICIENCY VIRUS EPIDEMIC.

wellness: Concept of experience dedicated to the principle that every individual, regardless of health status, can experience a heightened sense of well being and an optimized quality of life.

Western blot: A test used for analyzing protein antigens. Antigens are separated by changing the electrical potential (electrophoresis) and then transferred to a solid substance by blotting. The substance or membrane is incubated with antibodies. Enzymatic or radioactive techniques are then used to detect the bound antibodies. This method is very precise and is used for detecting small quantities of antibodies.

whey: Watery liquid that is a by-product of cheese production. A modified protein derived from whey blocked HIV infection of cells in vitro in a study conducted at the New York Blood Center and reported in *Nature Medicine.* Whey proteins may also be beneficial as a dietary supplement for seropositive individuals, helping to maintain or increase weight when combined with an adequate diet.

Whipple's disease: A malabsorption syndrome characterized by abnormal skin pigmentation, diarrhea, weight loss, weakness, arthritis, lymphadenopathy, and lesions of the central nervous system.

WHO: *See* WORLD HEALTH ORGANIZATION.

WIC: *See* WOMEN, INFANTS, AND CHILDREN.

will: (1) A legal statement of an individual's wishes concerning the disposal of his/her property after death. (2) The mental capacity for making a reasoned choice or decision. (3) The strength and power of controlling one's own actions.

window period: Period between infection with the human immunodeficiency virus and the appearance of antibodies to the virus in the bloodstream. The time can range from 2 weeks to 6 months.

Women, Infants, and Children (WIC): Operated through the Food and Nutrition Service of the *Department of Agriculture,* WIC is a federal grant program that targets low-income, nutritionally at risk, pregnant and lactating women, infants, and children up to age 5. WIC serves 45 percent of all infants born in the United States. The program is administered through state agencies and operated through various local agencies, including clinics and state and county health departments. Women, Infants, and Children, United States Department of Agriculture, 14th and Independence, S.W., Washington, DC 20250. Telephone: Using the Web site, look under the state or region for which information is desired. Full information, including telephone and fax numbers, is included. E-mail is also available directly from the Web site, <http://www.fns.usda.gov/wic/>.

Women's Bureau: Authorized by legislation in June 1920, the Women's Bureau is the only unit within the federal government that is exclusively concerned with serving and promoting the interests of working women. The Bureau is specifically mandated to advocate and inform both women and the public about women's work rights and employment issues. U.S. Department of Labor, Women's Bureau Office of Public Affairs, 200 Constitution Avenue, N.W., Room S-3311, Washington, DC 20210. Telephone: (202) 219-6652; Web site, <http://www.dol.gov/dol/wb/>.

works: Paraphernalia used by substance abusers for the illicit intravenous injection of drugs.

World Health Organization (WHO): Founded in 1948, this international organization is the health agency of the United Nations. Its goal is to achieve the optimum level of health care for all people. Objectives of the WHO include directing and coordinating international health work, ensuring technical cooperation, promoting research, preventing and controlling disease, and generating and disseminating information. The Organization emphasizes and supports the health needs of developing countries; establishes standards for biological, food, and pharmaceutical needs; and determines environmental health criteria. World Health Organization, 20 Avenue Appia, CH-1211 Geneva 27, Switzerland. Telephone: 41 22 7912111.

World Health Organization Collaborating Centre on AIDS: Founded in 1985 and now defunct, this health agency was chartered by the World Health Organization to conduct research and education and training programs concerning HIV and AIDS in order to promote public health. World Health Organization Collaborating Centre on AIDS, c/o Centers for Disease Control, 1600 Clifton Road NE, Atlanta, GA 30333. Telephone: (404) 639-3311.

World Health Organization Global Programme on AIDS: *See* JOINT UNITED NATIONS PROGRAM ON AIDS.

World Hemophilia AIDS Center: Founded in 1983, this organization functions as a clearinghouse for information concerning AIDS and hemophilia patients. The Center also collects data and conducts research to determine the extent of infection among hemophiliacs. World Hemophilia AIDS Center, 10 Congress Street, Suite 340, Pasadena, CA 91105. Telephone: (818) 577-4366.

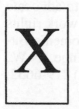

X ray: *See* RADIOGRAPHY.

Xanax: *See* ALPRAZOLAM.

xerosis: Abnormal dryness of the skin, mouth, or eyes.

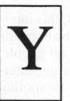

yeast: A general term including any of several unicellular, usually rounded, fungi that reproduce by budding. Some transform to a mold stage under certain environmental conditions, while others remain unicellular. A few yeasts are pathogenic in humans.

yeast infection: Invasion and multiplication of yeasts in body tissues that may produce injurious effects.

yellow dock: Herb used as an alternative therapy to treat various skin conditions—especially boils, rashes, and burns—and as an iron supplement for the treatment of anemia.

yellow nail syndrome: A syndrome associated with an excessive amount of fluids in the body tissues due to obstruction of the lymphatics, especially of the legs. The nails become yellowish to greenish in color; may be smooth, thickened, or excessively curved; slow in growth; and may become loose, causing them to be shed.

yin-yang: Concept of opposites, developed many centuries ago in China from observing the interdependent opposites in the physical world, like heat and cold. A fundamental tenet of Chinese traditional medicine teaches that when the yin and yang within each human body is in balance, good health is achieved; conversely, an imbalance of yin and yang in the body results in sickness.

Yodoxin: *See* IODOQUINOL.

yoga: Developed in the region that is now India, yoga is a system of techniques—including meditation and various postures—designed to enhance consciousness and to unify the individual consciousness to the universal one. Yoga postures maintain extraordinary flexibility in people who practice them throughout their lives.

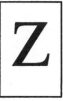

zalcitabine (ddC): First drug approved under the FDA's accelerated drug approval process, in 1992. It is a nucleoside analogue similar to zidovudine, but exhibiting less toxicity. The trade name is HIVID.

Zerit: *See* STAVUDINE.

Ziagen: *See* ABACAVIR.

zidovudine (AZT): A synthetic thymidine (one of the basic components of deoxyribonycleic acid) that inhibits the growth and development of the human immunodeficiency virus which causes the acquired immunodeficiency syndrome. It was the first antiretroviral therapy approved by the Food and Drug Administration. The trade name is Retrovir. *See also* THYMIDINE. *Also called* AZIDOTHYMIDINE.

zinc: Essential nutrient for all animals, as it functions in virtually all metabolic pathways in the body. Good dietary sources for zinc are meat, eggs, and seafood.

Zithromax: *See* AZITHROMYCIN.

Zofran: *See* ODANSETRON.

Zoloft: *See* SERTRALINE.

zoophilic sexual contact: Preference for sexual contact with animals rather than humans.

Zovirax: *See* ACYCLOVIR.

Appendix

Contact Information
for Governmental Entities
in the United States

Note: The federal government entities selected to appear in this appendix are those most likely to sponsor programs or provide information regarding HIV/AIDS. For a complete listing of governmental offices, refer to the most recent edition of the *U.S. Government Manual*. For a brief description of the work performed by the entity and further contact information, look in the text under the name of the agency.

Contact information provided in this Appendix is current as of May 2000.

Administration for Children and Families (ACF)
370 L'Enfant Promenade
Washington, DC 20447
Telephone: Staff and regional directories available on the Web site.
World Wide Web: <http://www.acf.dhhs.gov/>

Administration on Aging (AOA)
330 Independence Avenue, S.W.
Washington, DC 20201
Telephone: (202) 619-7501
TDD: (202) 401-7575
Fax: (202) 260-1012
Eldercare Locator: (800) 677-1116
World Wide Web: <http://www.aoa.dhhs.gov/>

Agency for Health Care Policy and Research (AHCPR)
Office of Health Care Information, Suite 501
Executive Office Center
2101 East Jefferson Street

Rockville, MD 20852
Telephone: (800) 358-9295
World Wide Web: <http://www.ahcpr.gov/>

Center for Information Technology (CIT)
National Institutes of Health
Building 12A, Room 1011
Bethesda, MD 20892
Information Office: (301) 496-6203
World Wide Web: <http://www.cit.nih.gov/>

Center for Mental Health Services (CMHS/SAMHSA)
P.O. Box 42490
Washington, DC 20015
Telephone: (800) 789-2647
TDD: (301) 443-9006
Fax: (301) 984-8796
World Wide Web: <http://www.mentalhealth.org/cmhs/index.htm>

Center for Scientific Review (CSR)
National Institutes of Health
6701 Rockledge Drive
Bethesda, MD 20892
Telephone: (301) 435-1099
World Wide Web: <http://www.csr.nih.gov/>

Center for Substance Abuse Prevention (CSAP/SAMHSA)
5600 Fishers Lane, Rockwall II
Rockville, MD 20857
Telephone: (301) 443-0365
World Wide Web: <http://www.samhsa.gov/csap/index.htm>

Center for Substance Abuse Treatment (CSAT/SAMHSA)
Telephone: (800) 662-4357 (Hotline for referrals for drug
    and alcohol treatment)
World Wide Web: <http://www.samhsa.gov/csat/csat.htm>

Centers for Disease Control and Prevention (CDC)
1600 Clifton Road
Atlanta, GA 30333
Telephone: (404) 639-3311; Toll-free, (800) 311-3435
World Wide Web: <http://www.cdc.gov/>

Child Nutrition
United States Department of Agriculture
14th and Independence, S.W.

Washington, DC 20250
World Wide Web: <http://www.fns.usda.gov/cnd/>

Civil Rights Division, Department of Justice
Office of the Assistant Attorney General
P.O. Box 65808
Washington, DC 20035
Telephone: (202) 514-2151
TDD: (202) 514-0716
Fax: (202) 514-0293
World Wide Web: <http://www.usdoj.gov/crt/>

**Criminal Section of the Civil Rights Division,
Department of Justice**
P.O. Box 66018
Washington, DC 20035
Telephone: (202) 514-3204
World Wide Web: <http://www.usdoj.gov/crt/>

Department of Agriculture (USDA)
14th and Independence, S.W.
Washington, DC 20250
Telephone: (202) 720-2791
TDD: (202) 720-2600
World Wide Web: <http://www.usda.gov/>

Department of Defense (DoD)
OASD (PA)/DPC
1400 Defense Pentagon, Room 1E757
Washington, DC 20301-1400
Telephone: (703) 697-5737
World Wide Web: <http://www.defenselink.mil/>

Department of Education (ED)
400 Maryland Avenue, S.W.
Washington, DC 20202
Telephone: (800) 872-5327
TTY: (800) 437-0833
Fax: (202) 401-0689
World Wide Web: <http://www.ed.gov/>

Department of Health and Human Services (DHHS)
200 Independence Avenue, S.W.
Washington, DC 20201

Telephone: (202) 619-0257; Toll-free: (877) 696-6775
World Wide Web: <http://www.dhhs.gov/>

Department of Housing and Urban Development (HUD)
451 7th Street, S.W.
Washington, DC 20410
Telephone: (800) 245-2691
World Wide Web: <http://www.hud.gov/>

Department of Justice
950 Pennsylvania Avenue, N.W.
Washington, DC 20530
World Wide Web: <http://www.usdoj.gov/>

Department of Labor (DOL)
Office of Public Affairs
200 Constitution Avenue, N.W.
Room S-1032
Washington, DC 20210
Telephone: (202) 693-4650
World Wide Web: <http://www.dol.gov/>

Department of the Treasury
Internal Revenue Service (IRS)
1111 Constitution Avenue, N.W.
Washington, DC 20024
Problem Resolution Hotline: (877) 777-4778
TDD: (800) 829-4059 (English/Spanish)
World Wide Web: <http://www.irs.ustreas.gov/>

Department of Veterans' Affairs (VA)
810 Vermont Avenue, N.W.
Washington, DC 20420
Telephone: (800) 827-1000
TDD: (800) 829-4833
World Wide Web: <http://www.va.gov/>

**Disability Rights Section of the Civil Rights Division,
Department of Justice**
P.O. Box 66738
Washington, DC 20035-6738
Telephone and TDD: (202) 307-0663
Fax: (202) 307-1198
World Wide Web: <http://www.usdoj.gov/crt/>

Drug Enforcement Administration (DEA)
Information Services Section (CPI)
700 Army-Navy Drive
Arlington, VA 22202
World Wide Web: <http://www.usdoj.gov/dea/>

Employment and Training Administration (ETA)
U.S. Department of Labor
ETA Office of Public Affairs
200 Constitution Avenue, N.W.
Room N-4700
Washington, DC 20210
Telephone: (202) 219-6871
World Wide Web: <http://www.dol.gov/dol/eta/>

**Employment Litigation Section
of the Civil Rights Division,
Department of Justice**
P.O. Box 65968
Washington, DC 20035
Telephone: (202) 514-3831
TDD: (800) 578-5404
Fax: (202) 514-1105
World Wide Web: <http://www.usdoj.gov/>

Equal Employment Opportunity Commission (EEOC)
1801 L Street, N.W.
Washington, DC 20507
Telephone: (800) 669-4000 (English/Spanish)
TDD: (800) 669-6820
World Wide Web: <http://www.eeoc.gov/>

Federal Bureau of Investigation (FBI)
J. Edgar Hoover Building
935 Pennsylvania Avenue, N.W.
Washington, DC 20353
Telephone: (202) 324-3000
World Wide Web: <http://www.fbi.gov/contact.htm>

Federal Mediation and Conciliation Service (FMCS)
2100 K Street, N.W.
Washington, DC 20427
Telephone: (202) 606-8100
Fax: (202) 606-4216
World Wide Web: <http://www.fmcs.gov/>

Federal Trade Commission (FTC)
CRC-240
Washington, DC 20580
Telephone: (202) 326-2000
World Wide Web: <http://www.ftc.gov/>

Food and Drug Administration (FDA)
FDA (HFE-88)
5600 Fishers Lane
Rockville, MD 20857
Telephone: (888) 463-6332
World Wide Web: <http://www.fda.gov/>

Food Stamp Program (FSP)
United States Department of Agriculture
14th and Independence, S.W.
Washington, DC 20250
Telephone: (800) 221-5689
World Wide Web: <http://www.fns.usda.gov/fsp/>

Health Care Financing Administration (HCFA)
Information Clearinghouse
7500 Security Boulevard
Baltimore, MD 21244
Telephone: (410) 786-3000
World Wide Web: <http://www.hcfa.gov/>

Health Resources and Services Administration (HRSA)
5600 Fishers Lane
Rockville, MD 20857
World Wide Web: <http://www.hrsa.dhhs.gov/>

HIV/AIDS Bureau of HRSA
Office of Communications
5600 Fishers Lane
Room 7-46
Rockville, MD 20857
Telephone: (301) 443-6652
Fax: (301) 443-0791
World Wide Web: <http://www.hrsa.dhhs.gov/hab/default.htm>

**Housing and Civil Enforcement Section
of the Civil Rights Division, Department of Justice**
P.O. Box 65998
Washington, DC 20035

Telephone: (202) 514-4713
Fax: (202) 514-1116
World Wide Web: <http://www.usdoj.gov/>

Indian Health Service
Communications Staff
Indian Health Service
Room 6-35, Parklawn Building
5600 Fishers Road
Rockville, MD 20857
Telephone: (301) 443-3593
Fax: (301) 443-0507
World Wide Web: <http://www.ihs.gov/>

John E. Fogarty International Center (FIC)
National Institutes of Health
Public Affairs Office
Building 31, Room B2C08
31 Center Drive, MSC 2220
Bethesda, MD 20892
Telephone: (301) 496-2075
Fax: (301) 594-1211
World Wide Web: <http://www.nih.gov/fic/>

Maternal AIDS Project
Director, Division of Advocacy and Special Issues
HCFA - Center for Medicaid and State Operations
7500 Security Boulevard
Baltimore, MD 21244
Telephone: (410) 786-1357
World Wide Web: <http://www.hcfa.gov/hiv/default.htm/>

Military Records Facility
9700 Page Avenue
St. Louis, MO 63132-5100
Telephone: (314) 538-4246
World Wide Web: <http://www.nara.gov/regional/stlouis.html/>

National Archives and Records Administration
700 Pennsylvania Avenue N.W.
Washington, DC 20408-0001
Telephone: (800) 234-8861
World Wide Web: <http://www.nara.gov/>

National Cancer Institute (NCI)
Office of Cancer Communications
31 Center Drive, MSC 2580
Bethesda, MD 20892
Telephone: (800) 422-6237 (English and Spanish)
TTY: (800) 332-8615
World Wide Web: <http://www.nci.nih.gov/>

**National Center for Complementary
and Alternative Medicine (NCCAM)**
NCCAM Clearinghouse
P.O. Box 8218
Silver Spring, MD 20907
Telephone: (888) 644-6226
TTY: (888) 644-6226
Fax: (301) 495-4957
World Wide Web: <http://nccam.nih.gov/>

National Center for Research Resources (NCRR)
Office of Science Policy
National Institutes of Health
Bethesda, MD 20892
Telephone: (301) 435-0888
World Wide Web: <http://www.ncrr.nih.gov/>

National Endowment for the Arts (NEA)
1100 Pennsylvania Avenue N.W.
Washington, DC 20506
Telephone: (202) 682-5400
World Wide Web: <http://www.arts.endow.gov/>

National Endowment for the Humanities (NEH)
1100 Pennsylvania Avenue N.W., Room 402
Washington, DC 20506
Telephone: (202) 606-8400
Fax: (202) 606-8240
World Wide Web: <http://www.neh.fed.us/>

National Eye Institute (NEI)
2020 Vision Place
Bethesda, MD 20892
Telephone: (301) 496-5248
World Wide Web: <http://www.nei.nih.gov/>

National Heart, Lung, and Blood Institute (NHLBI)
National Institutes of Health
Building 31, Room 5A03
31 Center Drive, MSC 2482
Bethesda, MD 20892
World Wide Web: <http://www.nhlbi.nih.gov/>

National Human Genome Research Institute (NHGRI)
National Institutes of Health
Building 31, Room 4B09
31 Center Drive, MSC 2152
Bethesda, MD 20892
World Wide Web: <http://www.nhgri.nih.gov/>

National Institute of Allergy and Infectious Diseases (NIAID)
Office of Communications and Public Liaison
Building 31, Room 7A-50
31 Center Drive, MSC 2520
Bethesda, MD 20892
Telephone: (301) 496-5717
World Wide Web: <http://www.niaid.nih.gov/>

**National Institute of Arthritis and Musculoskeletal
and Skin Diseases (NIAMS)**
National Institutes of Health
Building 31, Room 4C05
31 Center Drive, MSC 2350
Bethesda, MD 20892
Telephone: (301) 496-8188
Fax: (301) 480-2814
World Wide Web: <http://www.nih.gov/niams/>

**National Institute of Child Health
and Human Development (NICHD)**
National Institutes of Health
Building 31, Room 2A03
31 Center Drive, MSC 2425
Bethesda, MD 20892
Telephone: (800) 370-3943
World Wide Web: <http://www.nichd.nih.gov/>

National Institute of Corrections (NIC)
Administrative Offices
320 First Street, N.W.
Washington, DC 20534

Telephone: (202) 307-3106; Toll-free (800) 995-6423
World Wide Web: <http://199.117.52.250/inst/>

National Institute of Dental and Craniofacial Research (NIDCR)
National Institutes of Health
Building 31, Room 51349
31 Center Drive, MSC 2290
Bethesda, MD 20892
Telephone: (301) 496-4261
World Wide Web: <http://www.nidcr.nih.gov/>

National Institute of Diabetes and Digestive and Kidney Diseases (NIDDK)
Office of Communications and Public Liaison
Building 31, Room 9A04
Bethesda, MD 20892
Telephone: (301) 496-3583
World Wide Web: <http://www.niddk.nih.gov/>

National Institute of Environmental Health Sciences (NIEHS)
P.O. Box 12233
Research Triangle Park, Durham, NC 27709
Telephone: (919) 541-3345
World Wide Web: <http://www.niehs.nih.gov/>

National Institute of General Medical Sciences (NIGMS)
National Institutes of Health
45 Center Drive, MSC 6200
Bethesda, MD 20892
Telephone: (301) 496-7301
World Wide Web: <http://www.nigms.nih.gov/>

National Institute of Mental Health (NIMH)
NIMH Public Inquiries
6001 Executive Boulevard
Room 8184, MSC 9663
Bethesda, MD 20892
Telephone: (301) 443-4513
Fax: (301) 443-4279
World Wide Web: <http://www.nimh.nih.gov/>

National Institute of Neurological Disorders and Stroke (NINDS)
Office of Communications and Public Liaison
P.O. Box 5801
Bethesda, MD 20824
World Wide Web: <http://www.ninds.nih.gov/>

National Institute of Nursing Research (NINR)
National Institutes of Health
31 Center Drive
Room 5B10, MSC 2178
Bethesda, MD 20892
Telephone: (301) 496-0207
World Wide Web: <http://www.nih.gov/ninr/>

National Institute on Aging (NIA)
Public Information Office
Building 31, Room 5C27
31 Center Drive
Bethesda, MD 20892
Telephone: (301) 496-1752
World Wide Web: <http://www.nih.gov/nia/>

National Institute on Alcohol Abuse and Alcoholism (NIAAA)
National Institutes of Health
6000 Executive Boulevard
Willco Building
Bethesda, MD 20892
World Wide Web: <http://www.niaaa.nih.gov/>

National Institute on Deafness and Other Communication Disorders (NIDCD)
Office of Health Communication and Public Liaison
31 Center Drive, MSC 2320
Bethesda, MD 20892
Telephone: (301) 496-7243
TTY: (301) 402-0252
Fax: (301) 402-0018
World Wide Web: <http://www.nih.gov/nidcd/>

National Institute on Drug Abuse (NIDA)
National Institutes of Health
6001 Executive Blvd.

Bethesda, MD 20892
Telephone: (301) 443-1124
World Wide Web: <http://www.nida.nih.gov/>

National Institutes of Health (NIH)
Building 1, Room 344
1 Center Drive, MSC 0188
Bethesda, MD 20892
World Wide Web: <http://www.nih.gov/>

National Labor Relations Board (NLRB)
1099 14th Street N.W.
Washington, DC 20570
World Wide Web: <http://www.nlrb.gov/>

National Library of Medicine (NLM)
National Institutes of Health
8600 Rockville Pike
Bethesda, MD 20894
Telephone: (888) 346-3656
World Wide Web: <http://www.nlm.nih.gov/>

National Personnel Records Center
Civilian Records Facility
111 Winnebago Street
St. Louis, MO 63118-4199
World Wide Web: <http://www.nara.gov/regional/stlouis.html>

National Science Foundation (NSF)
4201 Wilson Boulevard
Arlington, VA 22230
Telephone: (703) 306-1234
TDD: (703) 306-0090
World Wide Web: <http://www.nsf.gov/>

NIC Information Center
1860 Industrial Circle, Suite A
Longmont, CO 80501
Telephone: (800) 877-1461 or (303) 682-0213
World Wide Web: <http://www.nicic.org/>

Occupational Safety and Health Administration (OSHA)
U.S. Department of Labor
OSHA Office of Public Affairs
200 Constitution Avenue, N.W.
Room N-3649

Washington, DC 20210
Telephone: (202) 693-1999
Emergency Line, for reporting a fatality or imminent
life-threatening situation: (800) 321-6742
World Wide Web: <http://www.osha.gov/>

Office of HIV/AIDS Policy
Hubert H. Humphrey Building
Room 730E
200 Independence Avenue, S.W.
Washington, DC 20201
Telephone: (202) 690-5560
Fax: (202) 690-7054
World Wide Web: <http://www.surgeongeneral.gov/
ophs/hivaids.htm>

Office of International and Refugee Health
Parklawn Building
Room 18-75
5600 Fishers Lane
Rockville, MD 20857
Telephone: (202) 443-1774
Fax: (202) 443-6288
World Wide Web: <http://www.surgeongeneral.gov/ophs/oirh.htm>

Office of Minority Health
Division of Information and Education
Rockwall II Building
Suite 1000
5600 Fishers Lane
Rockville, MD 20857
Telephone: (800) 444-6472 or (301) 443-5224
Fax: (301) 443-8280
World Wide Web: <http://www.omhrc.gov/>

Office of National AIDS Policy (ONAP)
736 Jackson Place
Washington, DC 20503
Telephone: (202) 456-2437
Fax: (202) 456-2438
World Wide Web: <http://www.whitehouse.gov/ONAP/>

Office of National Drug Control Policy (ONDCP)
Executive Office of the President
Washington, DC 20503

Telephone: (202) 395-6700
World Wide Web: <http://www.whitehousedrugpolicy.gov/>

Office of Public Health and Science (OPHS)
Assistant Secretary for Health, U.S. Surgeon General
Hubert H. Humphrey Building
Room 716G
200 Independence Avenue, S.W.
Washington, DC 20201
Telephone: (202) 690-7694
Fax: (202) 690-6960
World Wide Web: <http://www.surgeongeneral.gov/ophs/>

Office of Science and Technology Policy (OSTP)
1600 Pennsylvania Avenue N.W.
Washington, DC 20502
Telephone: (202) 395-7347
World Wide Web: <http://www.whitehouse.gov/
    WH/EOP/OSTP/html/OSTP_Home.html>

Office of Veterans Affairs and Military Liaison
Hubert H. Humphrey Building
Room 719H
200 Independence Avenue, S.W.
Washington, DC 20201
Telephone: (202) 260-0576
World Wide Web: <http://www.surgeongeneral.
    gov/ophs/ovaml.htm>

Office on Women's Health
U. S. Public Health Service
Department of Health and Human Services
200 Independence Avenue, SW
Room 730B
Washington, DC 20201
Telephone: (202) 690-7650
Fax: (202) 690-7172
World Wide Web: <http://www.4woman.gov/owh/>

Pension and Welfare Benefits Administration (PWBA)
U.S. Department of Labor
PWBA Office of Public Affairs
200 Constitution Avenue, N.W.
Room N-5656
Washington, DC 20210

Telephone: (202) 219-8921
World Wide Web: <http://www.dol.gov/dol/pwba/>

Social Security Administration (SSA)
Office of Public Inquiries
6401 Security Boulevard
Room 4-C-5 Annex
Baltimore, MD 21235
Telephone: (800) 772-1213
TTY: (800) 325-0778
World Wide Web: <http://www.ssa.gov/>

Substance Abuse and Mental Health Services Administration (SAMHSA)
5600 Fishers Lane
Rockville, MD 20857
Telephone: (301) 443-8956
World Wide Web: <http://www.samhsa.gov/>

U.S. Commission on Civil Rights (USCCR)
624 9th Street N.W.
Washington, DC 20425
Telephone: (202) 376-8312 (Public Affairs Unit)
World Wide Web: <http://www.usccr.gov/>

Veterans' Employment and Training Service (VETS)
U.S. Department of Labor
VETS Office of Public Affairs
200 Constitution Avenue, N.W.
Room S-1310A
Washington, DC 20210
Telephone: (202) 219-5573
World Wide Web: <http://www.dol.gov/dol/vets/>

Warren Grant Magnuson Clinical Center (CC)
National Institutes of Health
Bethesda, MD 20892
Telephone: (800) 411-1222
Fax: (301) 480-9793
World Wide Web: <http://www.cc.nih.gov/>

Women, Infants, and Children (WIC)
United States Department of Agriculture
14th and Independence, S.W.

Washington, DC 20250
World Wide Web: <http://www.fns.usda.gov/wic/>

Women's Bureau (WB)
U.S. Department of Labor
WB Office of Public Affairs
200 Constitution Avenue, N.W.
Room S-3311
Washington, DC 20210
Telephone: (202) 219-6652
World Wide Web: <http://www.dol.gov/dol/wb/>

T - #0511 - 101024 - C0 - 212/152/14 - PB - 9780789012074 - Gloss Lamination